DATE DUE

The Moral Challenge
of Alzheimer Disease

RECENT AND RELATED TITLES
IN GERONTOLOGY

John D. Arras, ed., *Bringing the Hospital Home: Ethical and Social
Implications of High-Tech Care*

Robert H. Binstock and Stephen G. Post, eds., *Too Old for Health
Care? Controversies in Medicine, Law, Economics, and Ethics*

Robert H. Binstock, Stephen G. Post, and Peter J. Whitehouse, eds.,
Dementia and Aging: Ethics, Values, and Policy Choices

Laurence B. McCullough and Nancy L. Wilson, eds., *Long-Term
Care Decisions: Ethical and Conceptual Dimensions*

Harry R. Moody, *Ethics in an Aging Society*

Robert H. Binstock, consulting editor in gerontology

The Moral Challenge
of Alzheimer Disease

STEPHEN G. POST

The Johns Hopkins University Press
Baltimore and London

The Johns Hopkins University Press
2715 North Charles Street
Baltimore, Maryland 21218-4319
The Johns Hopkins Press Ltd., London

Library of Congress Cataloging-in-Publication Data will be found
at the end of this book.
A catalog record for this book is available from the British Library.

ISBN 0-8018-5174-2

Contents

❧ Preface

As our aging population continues to grow older, the care of people with dementia, most often of the Alzheimer type, will severely test the moral fabric of the family and society. The moral basis of our commitment to those with significant progressive and irreversible loss of cognitive function must be reaffirmed and rearticulated. A new urgency of the ethics of dementia gives rise to this book, the first monograph on the topic but surely not the last.

Words are terribly limited; they can neither capture the ineffable depth of solicitude that shapes the caregiver experience nor convey the shaken existential foundations of the individual who confronts the journey into forgetfulness. But these limited words are at least neither abstract nor inaccessible, and they are informed as much as possible by attentive listening to affected families and individuals. If this book is worthwhile, it must be because it is written in the tradition of the public intellectual who wishes to convey ideas to a wide readership about matters of concern.

There are people to thank. Foremost, Joseph M. Foley, M.D., a much-loved patriarch of dementia care in Greater Cleveland and throughout the United States, not only introduced me to the moral problem of dementia but also has been a constant partner in conversation. His wisdom and care are deeply appreciated by me and by so many others. Peter J. Whitehouse, M.D., Ph.D., has continuously encouraged my involvement with the Alzheimer Center of University Hospitals of Cleveland and of Case Western Reserve University. Robert H. Binstock, Ph.D., has taught me much about gerontology and has been a faithful colleague. The Center for Biomedical Ethics of the Case Western Reserve University School of Medicine has served as an enriching intellectual environment. Harry R. Moody, Ph.D., deputy director of the Brookdale Center on Aging of Hunter College and an invaluable source of insight, suggested revisions in the manuscript that much improved its quality. But most of all, I owe thanks to the people with dementia and their families with whom I have had opportunity for dialogue through the facilitation of my friend Sharen K. Eckert, executive director of the Cleveland Area Chapter of the Alzheimer's Association.

This book was completed with the generous support of a grant from the Program on the Ethical, Legal, and Social Implications of Human Genome Research, National Institutes of Health (R01 HG0192-01A1). Additional support from the Cleveland Foundation was also helpful.

My wife, Mitsuko, my daughter Emma, and my son Andrew have often supported me in this endeavor, probably much more than they know. A note of thanks goes to my parents, Henry and Marguerite Post, who help us out in many ways. Thanks go, too, to St. Paul's School, in New Hampshire, where as a young student I first read Augustine on the meaning of memory.

ONE

ঈ Introduction:
Thinking about Forgetfulness

Seldom does human experience require more courage than in living with the diagnosis and the gradual decline of irreversible progressive dementia, most often of the Alzheimer type. While the body of the person with dementia will often remain strong for a number of years, mental capacities as well as the accumulated competencies and memories of a lifetime painfully slip away. This slippage is less emotionally traumatic for the affected individuals only when they begin to forget that they forget. Some people with Alzheimer disease (AD) live for two decades after initial clinical symptoms, although most live on for no more than seven or eight years. It is easy to understand why many fear dementia as much as or even more than cancer, for with cancer self-identity is usually not at stake, and physical pain can in most instances be controlled without compromising mental lucidity.

How can affected individuals and their caregivers maintain "the courage to be" before the foreboding specter of dementia? Among the several most urgent questions of our time is whether human beings have in place the moral and ethical signposts that can point toward a future in which those who are so forgetful will be treated with dignity (Binstock, Post, and Whitehouse, 1992). This book attempts to articulate these signposts, although words can neither fully express nor adequately honor the moral strength of caregivers and their loved ones. I can merely reflect on the emotionally wrenching stories of moral heroism as dementia breaks into the previously routine lives of individuals and families, like a huge wave disrupting everything in its path. The person with dementia is eventually swept away while caregivers look back and feel forever changed by their experiences.

My focus is on the elderly person with a progressive and irreversible dementia of the Alzheimer type, although Parkinson, Huntington, Pick, and Creutzfeldt-Jakob diseases are among the numerous non-Alzheimer causes of progressive dementia (Morris, 1994; Whitehouse, 1993). Dementia, which commonly refers to a precipitous decline in mental function from a previous state, can occur at any age, and may or may not be irreversible. For example, if AD is the dementia of elderly people, increasingly AIDS is the dementia of many who are relatively young (Clifford and Glicksman, 1994; Day et al., 1992). As our aging society continues a demographic transition in which those 85 and older constitute the fastest-growing age group, the numbers of elderly persons with chronic dementing diseases will reach a level of magnitude that human history has never before witnessed (Pifer and Bronte, 1986). There is potential for moral travesty or moral triumph. Because we have successfully eliminated many of the conditions that shorten the human life span, the thickness and thinness of our moral respect for elderly and debilitated persons takes on a new importance. The demands of filial morality and communal regard for elderly persons set forth in virtually all traditional social thought are now higher. Do we have the moral resources to navigate this crisis?

Moral Solidarity

This book calls for a critical reflection on cultural attitudes toward people with dementia, especially on the attitude that nothing can be done for them. Solidarity, comfort, and reassurance are not "nothing." A new ethics of dementia care will not accept the postulate of some ethicists that rationality and memory are the features of the person that give rise to moral standing and protection. Too great a value emphasis on rationality and memory, arguably the cardinal values of modern technological societies, wrongly excludes people with dementia from the sphere of human dignity and respect. Rationalistic theories of moral standing, of who counts under the protective canopy of "do no harm," discriminate against and unacceptably dehumanize those among us who most need our moral commitment because they are most forgetful. It is easy to be against people with dementia because our culture is against forgetfulness.

A respect for the whole person, and not for reason or memory alone, has classically been based on the assumption that the human being is sacrosanct. Will, emotion, and relational capacity counted as the morally relevant features of the person whose rationality and memory had faded. The myriad nursing homes sprinkled from coast to coast with roots in Protestant, Catholic, and Jewish traditions of care for the weak and vulnerable give testimony to the social importance of an ethics that refuses to condemn those who forget even their own names to a lowered tier of moral standing. The value of a human life rests not in reason and memory alone. Indeed, the weak of mind serve to confound the wise and mighty, disrupting the superficial sense that we human beings have full control over our fates and requiring that the sources of altruism within the self be discovered in the context of sometimes arduous care.

But we live in a culture that is the child of rationalism and capitalism, so clarity of mind and economic productivity determine the value of a human life. The dictum "I think, therefore I am" is not easily replaced with "I will, feel, and relate while disconnected by forgetfulness from my former self, but still, I am." Neither *cogito* (I think) nor *ergo* (therefore), but *sum* (I am). Human beings are much more than sharp minds, powerful rememberers, and economic successes. One of my colleagues, an epidemiologist who studies AIDS, tells the story of a young man with AIDS-related dementia who felt "written off" by his mentally agile friends. In response, he started a small business selling shirts with "Sum, I am" printed on them to people with AIDS. The key to an adequate ethics of dementia is full attention to the many ways of enhancing the noncognitive aspects of human well-being while not underestimating remaining capacities.

Rather than allowing declining mental capacities to divide humanity into those who are worthy or unworthy of full moral attention, it is better to develop an ethics based on the essential unity of human beings and on an assertion of equality despite unlikeness of mind. Instead of mirroring the inequalities of a hypercognitive culture, the ethics of dementia attaches no moral relevance to mental acuity or decline. The value of a human being is not diminished by even profound forgetfulness; we must assume equal moral seating and awaken a new beneficence toward those who can no longer remember.

I further think that full self-identity, made possible by an intact memory that connects past and present, should not be overvalued lest those who are disconnected from their pasts by forgetfulness be excluded from the protective canopy of "do no harm." Our ethics must respect those who, while unable to remember past events, still require emotional and relational well-being in the present. A common philosophical-existential emphasis on the self's "authenticity," defined as a consistent set of values and sense of self over an extended period of time, excludes those whose self is increasingly fragmented and scattered.

People with dementia have heterogeneous disabilities that confer on them a preferential moral significance based on the magnitude of their needs. They are the socially outcast, the unwanted, the marginalized, and the oppressed. A remarkable amount of elder abuse and neglect falls upon people with dementia, not just because caregivers are exhausted or ignorant, but because they are defenseless and easily victimized (Lucas, 1991).

It is morally relevant that according to some theorists, including Alois Alzheimer himself, dementia of the Alzheimer type may not fit the traditional disease model but is instead a threshold on the continuum of aging.

If the continuum model is correct, then we might all become severely demented if we live long enough, and we are all to some greater or lesser extent demented from the point in young adulthood when the human brain reaches its highest power (Huppert, Brayne, and O'Connor, 1994). Thus, the line blurs between "those" who are demented and "us" who are not. It is possible that social attitudes would change if we better appreciated the fact that we are all a little demented.

This is not a technical book, for the biomedical and social scientific aspects of dementia are covered in scores of other publications. While conversant with the sciences, I write as a humanist, ethicist, social philosopher, and at moments, a theologian. If successful, the book will contribute to thoughtfulness about people with dementia. There is nothing "soft" about thoughtfulness, as though only "hard" data count. Indeed, it is imperative that we now think hard about how to include people with dementia under the sacred canopy of "do no harm," despite the pressures of a hypercognitive culture to exclude.

We have not done enough to accept people with dementia into our midst. When Jonathan Swift described the demented "struldbrugs" in *Gulliver's Travels*, people with "no remembrance of anything but what they learned and observed in their youth and middle age, and even that is very imperfect," he indicated that "they are despised and hated by all sorts of people" (Swift, 1945, pp. 214–216).

The Ethics of Dementia: An Expanding Circle

Concern with dementia and ethics is inescapable in modern advanced nations, for the ranks of the gerontologist's "old-old," those 85 and older, are swelling as never before. There are currently nearly 4 million cases of AD in the United States; 9 million are projected by the year 2040. The most recent analysis indicates that the total cost of caring for an AD patient in northern California is approximately $47,000 per year whether the patient lives at home or in a nursing home. The total national cost for AD care is estimated at above $100 billion (Rice et al., 1993). In a culture that tends to abjure dependence, many older persons will not want to burden their families with the high cost of care. Moreover, it is altogether possible that in a culture that ultimately values productivity, the costs associated with AD care will not get very high priority. As families and as societies, we must struggle to be guided by moral principle despite economic strains; for professionals, dementia will become a major concern.

Why should dementia be of paramount concern for lawyers? Law is confounded by dementia. Ronald Dworkin, a preeminent philosopher of law, at the conclusion of a treatise on the interface of law and medicine, entitles his final chapter "Life Past Reason" (1993, p. 218). His words ring true: "We turn finally to what might be the saddest of the tragedies we have been reviewing. We must consider the autonomy and best interests of people who suffer from serious and permanent dementia" (Dworkin, p. 218). He notes that most persons with late-stage AD "still enjoy comfort and reassurance," and this is surely true (p. 229). Dworkin endorses "precedent autonomy" as genuine; that is, he argues that the medical decisions that the person expressed prior to becoming demented should be honored, even though that person has not yet experienced dementia. In the case of the person with severe dementia who is well adjusted emotionally and seems to be happy, Dworkin still endorses the authority of extended autonomy through advance directives such as living wills: "His former decision remains in force because no new decision by a person capable of autonomy has annulled it" (1993, p. 227).

While I agree with Dworkin's defense of precedent autonomy, there are others who view the AD-affected person in his or her present situation, and who are concerned only with current best interests regardless of previously expressed desires. While the indications of precedent autonomy, if now harmful and inhumane, should be overridden on the basis of current best interests, it is remarkable that some legal scholars seriously question precedent autonomy more generally, both conceptually and in application (Dresser, 1994). The issue is raised here only by way of introduction to underscore just how complex the ethical quandaries of dementia care are, including the questions of whether the "then" self should control the destiny of what gerontologists refer to as the "now" or demented self.

Why should dementia be of paramount concern for religious people and thinkers? For the theologian, the problem of dementia is urgent. How does one reconcile the decline of the demented self with the existence of a benevolent deity? Surely the AD-affected person confronts a slow taking away that rivals anything in the Book of Job, since Job was finally restored to prosperity. The evil of dementia cannot be placed at the door of human free will but in the sphere of the natural for which God is author. How could God allow this? Why do bad things happen to good people? Or is this even a coherent theological question (Hauerwas, 1990)? For the religious thinker, how can the notion of the soul, that permanent substratum of the self that exists in some ineffable continuity with the eternal, be thought to exist amidst such self-fragmentation? If the "soul" is the essence of the human personality, related to the body but more than a mere expression of the bodily and neurological because it includes possibilities beyond the order of time, what is the fate of this supposedly indestructible essence before the power of severe dementia (McNeill, 1951)? In November of 1993 a plenary session on theology and dementia was convened at the American Academy of Religion, attracting renowned scholars and an audience of hundreds.

Literature and drama also struggle to find some heuristic key into the meaning of dementia, or the lack thereof. Shakespeare's realistic and cynical Jacques from *As You Like It* proclaims: "Last scene of all, / That ends this strange eventful history, / Is second childishness and mere oblivion, / Sans teeth, sans eyes, sans taste, sans everything." Matthew Arnold's (d. 1888) poem "Growing Old" captures loss or radical diminution of powers, as do Balzac's (d. 1850) images of Pere Goriot (Bagnell and Soper, 1989). Two recent novels about the experience of dementia decline are Oliver Sacks's *Man Who Mistook His Wife for a Hat* and John Bernlef's *Out of Mind.* Literature pointing to the devastation of dementia is a necessary counterpoint to images of old age as a stage of wisdom and even of superiority to preceding stages.

Why should dementia be of paramount concern for economists and policymakers? In hard economic times, with health care rationing and intergenerational justice under discussion, how much will American society be willing to spend on the severely demented person (Binstock and Post, 1991)? Will compassion be too costly? Despite the cherished belief that no price tag can be put on a human life, can we afford to create state-of-the-art nursing homes for all dementia patients who need them? Will concerns with cost foster negative images of AD patients and encourage social decisions to limit life-extending treatment? The question of whether America can afford the booming elderly population is complicated by the high costs of good dementia care.

I raise these broad introductory questions to stress that dementia is a problem of the highest magnitude for all those who reflect on the human condition and the human future. But I do not consider dementia to be something we should merely think about, for then dementia ethics becomes more like an intellectual's game than a serious activity. Fortunately, while writing this book I had the opportunity to be steeped in the activities and concerns of the Alzheimer's Association chapter in Cleveland, in clinical settings, in the work of the Alzheimer Center of University Hospitals of Cleveland, and in the myriad programs at the Fairhill Center for Aging. Sprinkled throughout this book are the thoughts of others who spoke to me from their own experience of dementia or of giving care.

We must not accept Dworkin's unfounded assumption: "Do the demented have a right to dignity? Some demented people, particularly in the late stages of their disease, seem to have lost the capacity to recognize or appreciate indignity, or to suffer from it" (Dworkin, 1993, p. 234). We must remain agnostic with regard to the experience of indignity in the late stages, and therefore we can assume only that indignity is experienced and felt. The person with dementia is still a human being, and this being human is basis enough to demand that dignity be upheld.

Thinking of Leo

I recently visited an African American man in the inner city. Leo, 82 years old, was diagnosed with probable AD eight years ago. He was once a professional boxer and a machine worker, so his body remains strong, although he is no longer able to push away caregivers forcefully. Each day a health care aide visits, attending to the surgically implanted feeding tube and the catheter implanted into his bladder through an incision below the naval. The aide turns Leo over, bathes him, and changes the sheets, since he has recently become bedridden. His bodily firmness is in contrast with his mental decline. That Leo is bedridden is partly a relief to May, his sister and caregiver. Just a few months earlier, May would wake up some nights with the breeze blowing through the door—Leo used to wander at night and sometimes managed to open the lock.

The house stinks of dog urine (a huge guard dog dominates the first floor), the floors are old beaten plywood, and the windows are painted shut. The neighborhood is cut off from the manufacturing jobs that have long since disappeared. There is no furniture save an old sofa and a chair downstairs, and upstairs a shining hospital bed with medical fixtures needed for the feeding tube and catheter. I feel that Leo is captive to a strange combination of urban poverty and medical technology.

When I question May, she states that she never heard about withdrawing treatment, nor had Leo when he was still competent. State laws omit any reference to the condition of dementia (most state laws on death and dying address the "terminal condition" and the persistent vegetative state), thereby discouraging responsible choices to limit technology.

People with dementia brought on by diseases as varied as AD and AIDS, unless they are among the elite 15 percent of Americans with clear advance directives, are vulnerable to medicalized dying with tubes in every orifice, natural and unnatural. If it is the wisdom of nature that people with profound dementia forget how to swallow, if it was wise when Plato wrote that to the dying food "appears sour and is so," I wonder about our technological audacity and readiness to "play God" by inserting tubes.

But May asks me, "Well, wouldn't that be like killing?" And I suppose that many people in this urban African American ghetto would feel the same way. "Anyway, he don't do no one no harm." May is a good sister, but she is approaching 80 and no longer energetic. She also acknowledges her appreciation for Leo's monthly social security checks.

Leo seems to be emotionally adjusted to his condition and free from pain, although he is anxious to be reminded of who he is. His speech has recently become more difficult to understand (I am editing his words for the reader's benefit). His first question was an unclear "Who am I?" May answers in a kind and jovial voice, "What do you mean, you know who you are. You're Leo. You were a boxer. You're my brother." Leo inquires, "Boxer? Was I?" "Yes you were," responds May. "Where I am?" asks Leo. "In Cleveland, where you've been living for years," says May. "Mobile?" inquires Leo. "No, you were born in Mobile [Alabama], but now you're in Cleveland," states May. "Who am I?" repeats Leo. "What, you forgot again who you are? You're Leo, silly," May responds. "School, school. Who was my mama?" "Why you silly bones," answers May, "You know your mama was Leona, and she was my mama too, and you don't go to school." "Who am I?" Leo asks again. The cycle of questions, answers, and forgetfulness goes on like a litany. As conversation continues, I begin to see that Leo quite enjoys asking these questions. He seems to forget so completely that there is no obvious frustration on his part when he repeats what he has just asked a half minute ago, because every word is new. May's patience and kind voice seem to relieve any anxiety. She does simple but meaningful things, like touch his hand or pat his shoulder. Leo lives only in the "now."

It is difficult to imagine the solicitude of dementia care absent the concerned family, yet for many who are not yet old, the family has to some extent eroded. The implications of this erosion as the life span extends and debilitating chronic illness increases are worrisome (Post, 1993a, 1994).

People with dementia express emotion and respond to kindness; they respond to their environment with pleasure or fear; some carry on conversations of a sort; they can be treated in a manner that lessens the moments of terror that must accompany the sense of self-fragmentation. Simple expressions of reassurance do much good. May has a tone of voice that clearly soothes Leo. Thus, there are numerous ways to give meaningful care that can make the experience of dementia less frightening and inhumane.

The medicalized care of "doing to" is easier but often less called for than the basic interactional care of "being with." The French philosopher Gabriel Marcel wrote of care or love as "creative fidelity," "attentive listening," and "the mystery of presence." Care, building on the foundation of solicitude, includes joy, compassion, commitment, and respect: care rejoices in the existence of the person with dementia, although it need not strive to prolong that existence; care responds supportively to the needs of the person with dementia, although these needs may be largely emotional; care is loyal even as the loved one fades from the sphere of familiar self-identity and becomes almost unknowing and therefore unknown, but still remembered.

(The place to begin an ethics of dementia is not in moral abstractions, but in listening attentively to caregivers and affected persons as they participate in support groups and share experiences. This is an ethics grounded in concrete experience and meaningful solidarity. The philosopher Hegel remarked that there are two kinds of knowledge, knowledge in the abstract and knowledge in the concrete. He added that only the latter is real. Much can be learned by observing the remarkable solicitude and loyalty that many caregivers feel, despite insufficient support systems. Dementia ethics begins with an appreciation for noncognitive well-being and a willingness to engage remaining capacities and memory; it can only be discovered in praxis and dialogue; it must be practical rather than deductive, abstract, and game-like.

Creative Forms of Care

People with dementia require a social and moral creativity equal to that which has gradually arisen in the context of retardation. "Dementia," of course, refers to a mental decline from a previous state, while "retardation" refers to arrested development. Yet there is room for comparison, suggested by the fact that people with Down syndrome who live into their forties invariably manifest AD dementia (Berg, Karlinsky, and Holland, 1993).

What theologian and ethicist Stanley Hauerwas states about people with retardation could apply to people with dementia. People with retardation can receive "oppressive care, a kind of care based on the assumption that the retarded are so disabled that they must be protected from the dangers and risks of life" (Hauerwas, 1986, p. 162). Their capacities and agency are easily underestimated, so that they are to some extent trained to be retarded. Societies have struggled to receive people with retardation in ways that most allow them to flourish. The key to good care is not only to "do for" people with retardation, but to "be with" them, for a readiness to be with bridges a gap between us and them that is "not unbridgeable" (Hauerwas, 1986, p. 176). Many of us feel repulsed by people with retardation if we have not been around them much; experience and acculturation can help. We fear them because we do not know them. Can we be morally rich enough as a society that the well-being of people with retardation is enhanced? In religious traditions, of course, it is exactly the concern with the downtrodden and weak that is a special mark of moral excellence, and "people with retardation fit that description" (Hauerwas, 1986, p. 178).

In the case of AD and other dementias, the high expectations of elderly spouses for a "golden" retirement turn to despair, interrupting the best-laid plans. Like people with retardation, people with dementia can also receive oppressive care, a kind of care that protects from all risks while ignoring capacities to make choices and live actively, so that they are to a degree made to be more demented than they are. Communities struggle to respond to people with dementia in affirming and creative ways. To reiterate an important point, the medicalized "doing for" is in some respects easier than "being with" and bridging a gap between us and them.

One of the best examples of moral creativity in dementia care is the development of "special care units" (SCUs), which have proliferated across the country in recent years. We are now beginning to see the development of forms of care for people with dementia that counter the pervasive sense that nothing can be done for them. The emergence of these distinct sections in nursing homes designated for the care of people with more severe dementia is laudatory, even if such care is too expensive. SCUs vary in quality, but many allow for just the sort of efforts to enhance the noncognitive well-being of people with dementia that our culture easily overlooks. For this reason, it is necessary to create a dedicated and trained group of professional caregivers who, in a conducive and stimulating environment, can do for people with dementia what they deserve.

SCUs provide a setting in which functioning and the quality of life can be improved. Excess disability can be caused by such things as inappropriate caregiver responses to behavioral difficulties, a tendency to create dependency in personal care functions rather than to assist residents in performing functions themselves, lack of stimulation and exercise, polypharmacy and overuse of medications, and noises or other environmental factors that adversely impact the person with dementia.

A principle of SCUs is that individuals with dementia have residual strengths; for example, they often remember how to perform tasks they did earlier in life, giving them a sense of fulfillment. A man who was severely demented still remembered his boyhood task of carrying wood, and by walking with a bit of kindling in hand, his self-esteem and emotional state improved dramatically. Another principle of SCUs is that behaviors that appear meaningless may not be. Thus, the person who wanders may actually be searching for something or someone, and appropriate responses are possible. Also, SCUs encourage family members to be present to the extent that they wish. The best SCUs are designed by architects who attempt to provide appropriate visual, tactile, auditory, and physical stimulation without causing stimulation overload and consequent distress. Designs are intended to protect residents while maximizing ambulatory opportunities and independence. Cues are built into the interior design to help residents find their way around without feeling lost.

Six theoretical concepts for SCUs quoted below come from a report produced by the U.S. Congress Office of Technology Assessment (1992, pp. 17–21). The concepts are intended to bring greater uniformity of purpose into the varied SCU context:

1. Something can be done for individuals with dementia.
2. Many factors cause excess disability in individuals with dementia. Identifying and changing these factors will reduce excess disability and improve the individuals' functioning and quality of life.
3. Individuals with dementia have residual strengths. Building on these strengths will improve their functioning and quality of life.
4. The behavior of individuals with dementia represents understandable feelings and needs, even if the individuals are unable to express the feelings or needs. Identifying and responding to those feelings and needs will reduce the incidence of behavioral problems.
5. Many aspects of the physical and social environment affect the functioning of individuals with dementia. Providing appropriate environments will improve their functioning and quality of life.
6. Individuals with dementia and their families constitute an integral unit. Addressing the needs of the families and involving them in the individuals' care will benefit both the individuals and the families.

Applied to people with dementia in all contexts, these principles are a strong benchmark in the emergence of a new ethic of dementia care. The ideas that these principles articulate lie at the core of the ethics of dementia and can be extended to home care.

The Moral Task: Where No Techno-fix Is Imminent

We ought not to pretend that some magic bullet for dementia is on the horizon, even though the hope for a cure is vital and meaningful. Such hopes may be problematic if they divert attention from the central moral task of changing attitudes and providing forms of care that attend to the noncognitive aspects of the self.

One of the most important of all clinical issues is the introduction of experimental drugs that have questionable value in mitigating the progression of dementia. Tacrine, for example, is currently being marketed under the clever name "Cognex" (from *cognoscere*, to know), implying that it makes some change in the abilities of the dementia patient. Some families caring for an individual with dementia would give almost anything in the hopes of a few days of greater lucidity. Caregivers often want the opportunity to try any new antidementia medication, even if the evidence for it is only anecdotal. As one elderly man remarked, "I have been up to my ears in caring and diapers, so if there is anything hopeful, like tacrine, I want it." This perspective is understandable.

Joseph M. Foley, M.D., a former president of the American Society for Neurology who has long been appreciated for his pioneering work in dementia care by countless families in Greater Cleveland, points out that after major tacrine trials by Alzheimer research centers in the U.S., *"Parturient montes, nascitur musculus* (the mountains are in labor and a little mouse is born)" (Foley, 1993, p. 1). The results were equivocal. As Foley states, "If vitamin B^{12} in pernicious anemia or insulin in diabetes were to be given a 9.5 to 9.9 on a scale of 10, tacrine would seem to rate a 0.1 to 0.5. The reasonable conclusion was that it was a marginally effective drug at best" (1993, p. 1). Nevertheless, tacrine was approved by the Food and Drug Administration in early 1993 for use in people with dementia. There were pressures for approval from clinicians, advocates for people with dementia, and the pharmaceutical industry. Foley suggests that the advertising will not identify Cognex as marginally beneficial to useless and that many will want it in their desperation, perhaps just to feel that they are doing *something.* Costs for families are estimated at one to two thousand dollars annually, possibly eroding resources for respite or other forms of care. Physicians face the dilemma of whether or when to prescribe Cognex when it is demanded. They will also have to monitor the benefits, if any, in a particular case, and balance this against side effects, including potential liver toxicity (Foley, 1993).

Tacrine studies suggest a "modest" effect, but a better word would be "minimal." An impact of statistical significance may be clinically meaningless (Davis et al., 1992). There is reason for serious ethical concern when the two major double-bind studies of tacrine reach different conclusions on the drug's global clinical significance. Even the scant evidence for benefit in the more optimistic study is exceedingly minimal (Farlow et al., 1992). And yet influential media, such as the *U.S. News & World Report,* uses the caption "For some 40 percent of Alzheimer's sufferers, Cognex offers a reprieve" (Podolsky, 1992).

Hopefully we will, in our hypercognitive culture, use the scientific method to cure AD. But the advent of such a miracle may be slow in coming, since there is still much scientific debate about even the most basic biochemical and cellular aspects of AD. "They" may never have a technological fix, however much some of the effects of progressive dementia can be treated.

Thus, for the foreseeable future, dementia of the Alzheimer type requires a human moral response that attends to basic matters of dignity and well-being before the foreboding specter of quickly growing numbers of people with AD. An estimated 4 million Americans with AD will likely double in just two or three decades. On the one hand, this makes research into the basic science of AD terribly urgent and well worth considerable social investment; on the other hand, we must deal with the moral task that is before us.

Overview of the Chapters

This book does not begin with ethical quandaries, with competing reasons for choices x and y in a specific medical case. Only the second half of the book attends to medical choices and analysis of arguments. Although medical and medicalized ethics are vitally important, my interest is much wider than this. Because the experience of people with dementia, many of whom will say that they do not wish to be called "patients," is much more than medical, the book opens with a discussion of this experience based largely on autobiographical narratives, and then takes up the most foundational questions of all—what is the moral significance of people with dementia? and how do cultural undercurrents diminish that significance? Thus, chapter 2 is entitled "Dementia, Discourse Ethics, and Well-Being" and chapter 3 is entitled "The Challenge of Respect and Beneficence." Legitimate disagreements about issues such as life prolongation and termination of treatment must wait for later chapters. Discussion of these disagreements, however, is much enhanced by these earlier considerations of experience and moral significance. Those who wish to press immediately into the quandaries of medical choice are urged to be patient, for the prior questions are necessary to set the background.

Chapter 4, "Familial Caregiving and the Ethics of Behavior Control," deals with the moral basis of caregiving by spouses and adult children of AD-affected individuals. Since familial caregiving is an important moral resource, it should not be exhausted but instead should be supported. Because the tasks of caregivers are often made arduous by behavioral difficulties in the person with dementia, the long-term best interests of the individual and of his or her caregivers are not easily separated. Thus, the ethics of behavior control must be linked to the preservation of the family as a context for caregiving.

The fifth chapter is methodologically unique because it is the fruit of a major community dialogue with AD-affected individuals, their family caregivers, and a group of interprofessional and interdisciplinary individuals concerned with dementia care. The chapter is shaped by consensus statements emerging from nine months of dialogue and focus-group activity. Here the book gets into the various quandaries that emerge with the chronology of progressive dementia, including diagnostic disclosure, limitations on driving and other activities, living wills and other forms of advance directive, and withdrawal of treatment including artificial nutrition and hydration.

Chapter 6 takes up the limelight issue of presymptomatic testing for AD and other dementias. The title of this chapter, "Presymptomatic Testing: An Amniocentesis for Elderly Persons," indicates my concerns with the cultural forces that drive elderly people toward testing and thereby increasingly medicalize their old age. I deal with both psychological and genetic testing designed to detect dementia in the preclinical stages.

The seventh chapter takes up a debate that has been ongoing and acrimonious for three decades, that is, the ethics of the quality of life versus the ethics of the sanctity of life. I attempt to construct a useful dialectic between quality and sanctity that does not discriminate against people with dementia but neither does it allow for the inhumane imposition of medical technology. This chapter is entitled "Quality of Life, Treatment Burdens, and the Right to Comfort." I might have included the right to reassurance.

The final chapter, "Dementia, Assisted Suicide, and Euthanasia," expresses cautions regarding the implementation of policies allowing preemptive assisted suicide and mercy killing for people with the diagnosis of probable AD. Like abortion, this is an area in which well-intentioned and conscientious people can meaningfully disagree. This chapter connects the debate with the issues of moral significance and cultural bias that form the nucleus of the first several chapters, thereby bringing the book to a coherent closure.

People with AD and other dementias, in addition to vital physical needs for safety, medical care, and nutrition, also have needs for stimulation, reassurance, companionship, and respect. Their needs are not categorically different from the needs of many very old people, although the degree of need is generally greater. Some societies have practiced senicide in the past, abandoning demented elderly people to the elements, rather than meeting these needs. The nonvoluntary euthanasia of elderly persons with dementia occurred in Germany between 1939 and 1941 under the ethic of "life unworthy of life." These realities are worth mentioning because unless we strive now to make innovative space for people with dementia in our society, the future may be less than progressive. How much moral progress can be made in the area of dementia ethics in any period of human history is an open question.

TWO

❧ Dementia, Discourse Ethics, and Well-Being

Because our culture so values rationality and productivity, observers easily characterize the life of the person with dementia in the bleakest terms because it lacks such sociocultural worth. The experience of the person with irreversible and progressive dementia is clearly tragic, but it need not be interpreted as half empty rather than as half full.

If we are to progress in the ethics and care of people with dementia, it is important to leap beyond narrow and negativizing assumptions into a purely descriptive appreciation for the individual and highly heterogeneous experience of the AD-affected person. By direct attention to the experience of dementia, it is possible to establish an ethics of respect for the subjectivity and dignity of those affected. Toward this end, the chapter proceeds, after a brief warning against what I shall call "exclusionary ethics," to narratives of the experience of dementia and noncognitive forms of well-being.

Exclusionary Ethics

The fitting response to the increasing incidence of dementia in our aging society is the enlargement of our sense of human worth to counter an exclusionary emphasis on rationality, efficient use of time and energy, ability to control distracting impulses, thrift, economical success, self-reliance, "language advantage," and the like. It is troubling that some moral philosophers base moral standing on currently operative capacities that seem to especially exclude people with dementia. Peter Singer, for example, cited approvingly a list of morally significant capacities or "indicators of personhood," that is, "self-awareness, self-control, a sense of the future, a sense of the past, the capacity to relate to others, concern for others, communication, and curiosity" (Singer, 1993, p. 86). Some of these capacities, which would give a right to moral and legal protection, are particularly lacking in people with moderate and advanced dementia, who therefore fail to fulfill the definition of "personhood." On Singer's behalf, he asserts equality as a moral principle relevant to the alleviation of suffering even for "nonpersons," but he still defends infanticide, and nonvoluntary killing of demented "nonpersons" does not trouble him (p. 192).

Critics of the "personhood" theories of ethics, among whom I must be included, think that a task of ethics is to include rather than exclude the vulnerable. The restricted definition of person has the consequence that some people are not persons and therefore do not count. Better to quicken the spirit of beneficence toward the mentally weakened rather than undermine it. Historically, this quickening is related to a shift in the moral tone of Western civilization that even gives preference to the vulnerable and weak and that makes beneficent service the highest virtue. This shift, which occurs in the early medieval period, is associated by the moral historian Lecky and by philosopher Charles Taylor with the process of western Christianization (Lecky, 1955; Taylor, 1989).

David H. Smith has pointed to the implications of the "personhood" revolt against inclusivity. He described the loyal care provided for his mother-in-law, Martha. A woman from an apartment down the hall from Martha called to say that she was getting lost and behaving strangely. Smith noted, however, that despite AD, "social graces remained: smiling at a visitor, laughing with the crowd, responding briefly and politely in conversation" (Smith, 1992, p. 45). Reflecting on several years of caring for Martha before her death (in a deep coma following a seizure), Smith raised the question of "identity, status, or ontology. How much do demented persons matter, and why do they matter?" (1992, p. 46). This is the seminal question that must be answered before all others.

Smith rejected the notion that "personhood," the basis of moral status, is measured by continuing moral agency. He cited biomedical ethicist H. Tristram Engelhardt Jr., who argues that people "are persons . . . when they are self-conscious, rational, and in possession of a minimal moral sense." By this narrow definition of personhood, Martha had ceased to be a person. Smith asked, "But what follows? That she need no longer be respected? That she was no longer part of the family? That it was incoherent to continue to love her? That she could make no reasonable claim on the resources or forbearances of the larger society?" (1992, p. 47). Smith's conclusion is that the narrow personhood theory of moral status is an "engine of exclusion" that can lead to "insensitivity" if not "wickedness."

The fundamental moral commitment of a good society is to protect all human beings, based not on their varied and unreliable capacities but on a radical human equality. Such equality in moral standing and consideration is easily broken by the power of the cognitively privileged as they demand additional privileges. The privileged are prone to create excessively rationalistic criteria for moral inclusion under the protective umbrella of "do no harm" and are confounded by loyalty to those whose minds have faded.

Coming Closer

I begin this ethics of dementia not with theories of "personhood" but with attentive listening to the voices of people with dementia. Their stories call us into the lived realities of dementia so that we then have something substantial about which to reflect. These narratives can affect and shift one's image of people with dementia so that ethical analysis is transformed.

Andrew D. Firlik described his encounters as a first-year medical student with a 55-year-old woman named Margo, diagnosed with AD (1991). As he wrote, "I crossed the street. I became close to Margo." Visiting her each day, he noticed that Margo "could listen to songs over and over, each time with the same enthusiasm as before." She could not recall his name, but she always greeted him graciously, "as if she had at least a general sense of who I am." Margo still loves peanut butter and jelly sandwiches. Despite her AD, "Margo is undeniably one of the happiest people I have known. There is something graceful about the degeneration her mind is undergoing, leaving her carefree, always cheerful" (p. 201). Firlik was obviously astounded and changed by his experiences. Clearly not many people with AD dementia adjust to forgetfulness as well as Margo did, and in some instances the experience is anything but this benign.

It is necessary to come closer to people with AD to overcome hypercognitive acculturation and unduly negativized stereotypes. It is also necessary to come closer to construct an ethics of liberation, which means to clarify and organize the voices of people with dementia and their caregivers consistent with the method of "discourse ethics" (Habermas, 1990, 1993). Discourse ethics represents a shift away from heavy reliance on ethical theory, although without abandoning basic moral principles such as "do no harm," beneficence, and respect for autonomy (self-determination). Such an ethics allows the process of dialogue with those who have dementia and their caregivers to define what aspects of the illness are morally important. It represents a deemphasis on the formal professionalized canons of ethics.

Discourse ethics was initially defined by the German political philosopher Jurgen Habermas. According to Habermas, moral norms do not derive from theory nor do they emerge from the solitary thinker; rather, they emerge as socially necessary dialogic creations that are universal insofar as they are agreed to by the community through authentic conversation, that is, with all participants at equal seating. Moral norms of universal value cannot easily emerge from solitary individuals because their "pure reason" is always their own and therefore grounded in a personal history with all its cultural biases and interests. Especially in grappling with the ethics of dementia, those who make an idol of reason may demonstrate a proclivity to exclude. They do not yet appreciate the redeeming words, "I am."

Experiencing the Anxiety of Forgetfulness

Beneficence can be quickened by recognizing and responding to the anxiety of those whose memories are fading. Before persons with dementia reach extreme self-forgetfulness, there is a period that may last for several years during which they depend on structures of meaning to make sense of their condition, sometimes against a religious background. People with dementia are meaning seeking in the same way that we all are, and their struggles to make sense of loss are akin to our own.

To present the picture of people with dementia as meaning seeking, I will rely on autobiographical accounts. The following story—only lightly edited—was told by a woman in her mid-40s with dementia, etiology unknown. Jan is conversant, although there are some days when she is too mentally confused to engage in much dialogue. She has more difficulty responding to open-ended questions but does very well if her conversation partner cues her by mentioning several alternative words from which she might choose, at which point she can be quite articulate.

It was just about this time three years ago that I recall laughing with my sister while in dance class at my turning the big 40. "Don't worry, life begins at forty," she exclaimed and then sweetly advised her younger sister of all the wonders in life still to be found. Little did either of us realize what a cruel twist life was proceeding to take. It was a fate neither she nor I ever imagined someone in our age group could encounter.

Things began to happen that I just couldn't understand. There were times I addressed friends by the wrong name. Comprehending conversations seemed almost impossible. My attention span became quite short. Notes were needed to remind me of things to be done and how to do them. I would slur my speech, use inappropriate words, or simply eliminate one from a sentence. This caused not only frustration for me but also a great deal of embarrassment. Then came the times I honestly could not remember how to plan a meal or shop for groceries.

One day, while out for a walk on my usual path in a city in which I had resided for eleven years, nothing looked familiar. It was as if I was lost in a foreign land, yet I had the sense to ask for directions home.

There were more days than not when I was perfectly fine; but to me, they did not make up for the ones that weren't. I knew there was something terribly wrong and after eighteen months of undergoing a tremendous amount of tests and countless visits to various doctors, I was proven right.

Dementia is the disease, they say, cause unknown. At this point it no longer mattered to me just what that cause was because the tests eliminated the reversible ones, my hospital coverage was gone, and my spirit was too worn to even care about the name of something irreversible.

I was angry. I was broken and this was something I could not fix, nor to date can anyone fix it for me. How was I to live without myself? I wanted Jan back!

She was a strong and independent woman. She always tried so hard to be a loving wife, a good mother, a caring friend, and a dedicated employee. She had self-confidence and enjoyed life. She never imagined that by the age of 41 she would be forced into retirement. She had not yet observed even one of her sons graduate from college, nor known the pleasures of a daughter-in-law, or held a grandchild in her arms.

Needless to say, the future did not look bright. The leader must now learn to follow. Adversities in life were once looked upon as a challenge; now they're just confusing situations that someone else must handle. Control of *my life* will slowly be relinquished to others. I must learn to trust—completely.

An intense fear enveloped my entire being as I mourned the loss of what was and the hopes and dreams that might never be. How could this be happening to me? What exactly will become of me? These questions occupied much of my time for far too many days.

Then one day as I fumbled around the kitchen to prepare a pot of coffee, something caught my eye through the window. It had snowed and I had truly forgotten what a beautiful sight a soft, gentle snowfall could be. I eagerly but so slowly dressed and went outside to join my son, who was shoveling our driveway. As I bent down to gather a mass of those radiantly white flakes on my shovel, it seemed as though I could do nothing but marvel at their beauty. Needless to say, he did not share in my enthusiasm; to him it was a job, but to me it was an experience.

Later I realized that for a short period of time, God granted me the ability to see a snowfall through the same innocent eyes of the child I once was, so many years ago. I am still here, I thought, and there will be wonders to be held in each new day; they are just different now.

Quality of life is different to me now from the way it was before. I am very loved, in the early stages, and now my husband and my sons give back in love what I gave them. I am blessed because I am loved. That woman who killed herself, you know, with that suicide doctor. She didn't have to wind up that way. Not that I condemn her, but our lives can't really be that bad. Her choice is understandable if she wasn't loved or cared for. Now my quality of life is feeding the dogs, looking at flowers. My husband says I am more content now than ever before! Love and dignity, those are the keys. This brings you back down to the basics in life; a smile makes you happy.

This woman experiences frustration, fear, loss of control, and anger, but she is able to adjust to her circumstances with some success. In my conversation with her, she emphasized two key factors that make adjustment possible. First, her husband discusses with her any limitations on her privileges, and she is able to reach consensus on safety issues. For example, she no longer drives, but on the condition that family members provide her with transportation. She no longer walks across the street alone because she is confused about the meaning of the red, yellow, and green lights, but this is on the condition that others escort her routinely. Second, she refers to the love she feels from her family and considers it essential to her quality of life.

I refer the reader to one of the better published autobiographical accounts from a person with Alzheimer disease. Robert Davis, a minister, found peace in his perception that his condition was a test of faith like Job's. But later, in more confused moments, even this theological framework was lost and he experienced profound anxiety and forsakenness, a shaking of all his foundations. His hope was for an imminent death to take him quickly rather than experience further loss of cognition and self-control.

In this account by a man trying to find meaning in subtle and then more dramatic changes occurring in his fading mind, the story of the disease is conveyed from the inside. The existential (or "gut level") story must be told powerfully for people without dementia to properly appreciate the struggle: "My brain may be dying, but in my spirit Christ has healed me, and I can say with the songwriter, 'It is well with my soul'" (Davis, p. 68). Later, "The private emotional relationship with the Lord that I enjoyed is distorted and does not comfort me now. When I pray, I often pray in silent blackness of spirit" (p. 110). He became periodically forgetful even of a cherished system of meaning to which his life was devoted. But in the last analysis, his faith, coupled with the support of his wife, Betty, allowed him to gain enough perspective on his condition to write a meaningful book with her help.

These accounts of dementia highlight individuals' endeavors to retain hope and meaning. Both remain persons, with their gratifications and frustrations, their own unique background, and their own unique destiny. There is a relatively benevolent point in the progression of dementia when all anxiety and embarrassment are forfeited in favor of amnesia. Family and friends become as strangers, while the familiar and the foreign lose the elasticity of their boundaries and become one (Buchanon, 1989). The mind fades to the point where one is no longer able to worry about this fading.

When the capacity to seek meaning in the midst of decline itself gives way to more advanced dementia, as it will in the more severe stages of illness, then the experience of the person must be understood in relational and affective terms rather than cognitive ones. Here the challenge to set aside the values of hypercognitive culture is upon us, and "personhood" ethics become dangerous.

Honoring the Faded Self

People with progressive dementia come to forget that they forget, and their anxiety over forgetfulness ceases. At a meeting with representatives from the local Alzheimer's Association (a support group for AD-affected individuals and their families), I conducted a discussion of the moral meaning of quality of life in the context of severe dementia. The group expressed much concern that only people with AD and their family caregivers are in a position to speak fairly about the quality of life. One caregiver said that it would be better to speak of the quality of lives, since the person affected with AD is not an individual but a loved one in essential relationship with spouse. While a later chapter is devoted to the ethical debate over dementia and the quality of life, the following anecdotes are offered here to further introduce the reader to the experience of dementia and its complexity.

Sharen's Father. Sharen told the story of her father. He held on to his identity until the very end, she said. He wore his favorite cowboy hat in the shower, slept with it on his head, and never let it out of his sight, even after entering the nursing home. Somehow he knew that there was something special about this hat, that it was somehow connected with who he was. While he could no longer talk much, and never coherently, he could still play a pretty good game of pinochle long after he forgot Sharen's name. "He never read books much anyway," remarked Sharen. "He worked in the steel mills and had lots of male drinking friends. People of intellectual capabilities would not have appreciated Dad's many moments of joy. Of course, there were down moments for Dad, like there are for everyone. But his quality of life cannot be adequately evaluated by the intellectuals, who are not a jury of his peers."

The moral of Sharen's account is that in her father's case, something of permanence in the self seems to have been retained, if his clutching his favorite old cowboy hat conveys anything meaningful. Sharen certainly found the hat to be a symbol of some underlying permanence.

Henry. My wife, Ruth, was told she had probable AD. She appreciated this because it gave her something to hang her hat on. She could tell people that she was ill and that she couldn't help her forgetfulness. We accelerated plans for travel, traveling all around the United States. Ruth especially loved the fall colors in New England and the ranches in Texas. In the nursing home, we still traveled in a way by walking around the wooded paths surrounding the home. Ruth used to whistle at birds, and I sometimes felt that they really understood her. She would gaze at a colorful flower for ten or fifteen minutes, all the time with a smile. Sometimes, with fractured words and sentences, she would say, "I love you." She still recognizes me, but not our 30-year-old daughter, although she has glimmers of recognition of her. Ruth spontaneously whistles, and she is able to keep time with music. She likes only soft music now. When she is agitated music can help. She still smiles a lot. A touch on the arm from a friendly person is always well received. The key is what the person with AD feels is quality of life, and we have to work at that level. Her response to music is declining now. How much should we try to restore her health? I oppose feeding tubes. As Ruth declines more, I want to withhold feeding. She will have to be moved to another nursing home that allows this. The goal is comfort, not life prolongation. She still knows who I am, she feels me, and she still loves me.

Mrs. G. Mrs. G. came from an old family of distinction. I visited her in the Alzheimer wing of a good-quality nursing home. She carries an old book under one arm as she walks slowly down the corridor. I greet Mrs. G., but she says nothing. However, she shows a picture to me and seems to smile, but I am not quite certain of this. It is a James Audubon print book. They tell me she always has it open to the same page and points to the same picture, a bluebird. (I think a bit sardonically that at least with dementia novelty requires only one book and one picture.) I guide Mrs. G. to a table and we sit. I ask her how her children are. She does not respond, although she again appears to smile. She seems to say "sky," but who knows?

She has a certain graceful charm and a slight smile. They say that habitual mannerisms and demeanor are so ingrained that they are the last things to go. Are these graces just the simulacrum of the self, a kind of deception that suggests more of Mrs. G. is there than meets the eye? Slowly Mrs. G. arises and walks away, a little tear in her eye. She seems to have emotions left, and emotions are a part of well-being. The ability to experience emotions has not been lost, and in this sense Mrs. G. is as fully human as anyone else, or even more so.

Because of the human propensity to treat with indignity those who supposedly cannot experience indignity, it is vital to assume a continuing self-consciousness and a correlative sensitivity to the manner of treatment afforded by others.

Last Tango in Paris. There is a story about Mrs. S. and Mr. R. Mrs. S. is now just past a stage of dementia in which behavioral abnormalities such as delusion and hallucination are commonplace in some patients. A nurse aide tells me about her. A year back, when Mrs. S. was hallucinating and more difficult to care for, she projected her long-since deceased but very much beloved husband's image on another resident in the Alzheimer unit, Mr. R. She managed to convey her affection to this gentleman, who was mildly to moderately demented himself and therefore capable of some insight. Mrs. S. would bring him any object she could reach for and make of it a gift. The old gentleman was thrilled.

On one of his better days—and patients fluctuate in the moderate stages—Mr. R. managed to ask the doctor if he might cohabit with Mrs. S. This was to be an old man's last tango in Paris, his final and ultimate hope. It appeared that Mrs. S. might have enjoyed this as well. The doctor took the request to the administration, which in turn took it to Mrs. S.'s adult daughter. The daughter was appalled at the request. Had not her mother and father loved each other for decades? Had they not been faithful and devoted to their marriage? Cohabitation makes a mockery of fidelity, nursing home ombudsperson be damned! No, Mrs. S. would be demeaned by intimacy with another man, himself demented and loved only on the basis of being mistaken for a dead spouse. So the nursing home administrator broke the bad news to the old man. No last tango; she thinks you are someone you're not. She mistook you for her husband. She sometimes mistakes people for coat racks.

The old man did not understand. He became increasingly depressed as the days wore on. He stopped talking and eating. He no longer wandered about. The staff put a feeding tube down his throat. After two months, the old man was moved to another nursing home. Several months later, with a feeding tube surgically implanted in his abdomen, he died of pneumonia. His family said it would be wise to let him die. No antibiotics were given. The nurses said that this was one case where an old man died of despair.

The quandary, of course, is whether the utilitarian norm of maximizing happiness should have been applied to this elderly woman and her prospective partner, allowing cohabitation on the assumption that the marital values of the precedent and intact self are no longer morally determinative. My undergraduate students, incidentally, have almost invariably sided with happiness.

Enhancing the Well-being of People with Dementia

Thus far in this chapter, I have attempted to bring the reader closer to the experience of dementia through dialogue with those who have struggled with profound forgetfulness. This is itself a part of discourse ethics, since without these stories there would be nothing concrete about which to reflect. As the philosopher Hegel insisted, there is only knowledge in the concrete, for knowledge in the abstract is not real. Discourse ethics builds on the concrete and should lead to more concern with the well-being of people with dementia and to a better understanding of the emotional dimension of that well-being.

Although those distant from the experience of dementia and not in discourse with affected people may find it difficult to imagine, Tom Kitwood and Kathleen Bredin developed a description of the "culture of dementia." They described twelve indicators of well-being in people with severe dementia: the assertion of will or desire, usually in the form of dissent despite various coaxings; the ability to express a range of emotions; initiation of social contact (for instance, a person with dementia has a small toy dog that he treasures and places it before another person with dementia to attract attention); affectional warmth (for instance, a woman wanders back and forth in the facility without much sociality, but when people say hello to her she gives them a kiss on the cheek and continues her wandering); social sensitivity in the form of a smile or taking another's hand; self-respect (for instance, a woman who has defecated on the floor in the sitting room attempts to clean up after herself); acceptance of other dementia sufferers (for instance, a fast wanderer takes the hand of a slow wanderer and leads him around); humor (as in the case of a technical problem with a video system when a person with severe dementia unexpectedly blurts out, "Try putting a shilling in the slot"); creativity and self-expression, often achieved through art or music therapy; showing evident pleasure through smiles and laughs in an exercise event; helpfulness (as in the case of a man who provided a cushion for a woman seated on the hard floor); and relaxation (for instance, one person with dementia takes the hand of another with a habit of lying on the floor curled up tensely and leads her to the sofa, where she relaxes) (Kitwood and Bredin, 1992, pp. 281–282). These indicators "are virtually independent of the complex cognitive skills that most adults continuously employ," but they have tremendous importance and validity (Kitwood and Bredin, 1992, p. 282). The goal of dementia care ethics is to enhance well-being through facilitating a sense of personal worth, a sense of agency, social confidence, and a basic trust or security in the environment and in others (Kitwood and Bredin, 1992, p. 283).

Some of those people "written off" as hopelessly demented may, given proper environmental and social cooperation, demonstrate a degree of temporary reversal, and perhaps with the proper creative activities the deterioration can be somewhat slowed (Kitwood and Bredin, 1992, p. 278). If so, caring is best construed not as the onerous supervision of decline but rather as a process of helpful interaction that mitigates the progression of dementia through enhancing well-being. The subjectivity of the person with dementia must be affirmed, including gestures and utterances as expressive of felt needs. It is wrong to underestimate what those with dementia can do with proper facilitation (Kitwood, 1993).

Discourse and the Moral Commitment to Communication

Part of discourse ethics is a commitment to special techniques of communicating with people with dementia in the hope of drawing on their remaining capacities. Ripich and Wykle (1990) have designed a program for enhancing communication between nurse aides and people with AD. This seven-step program uses the acronym FOCUSED to identify the major elements for the maintenance of communication (Face-to-face, Orientation, Continuity, Unsticking, Structure, Exchanges, and Direct). The program is based on an interactive discourse model of conversational exchanges.

The strategies used to accomplish FOCUSED communication maintenance with AD-affected individuals are the following:

F = Face to face:
    1. Face the person directly.
    2. Attract the person's attention.
    3. Maintain eye contact.
O = Orientation:
    1. Orient the person by repeating key words several times.
    2. Repeat sentences exactly.
    3. Give the person time to comprehend what you say.
C = Continuity:
    1. Continue the same topic of conversation for as long as possible.
    2. Prepare the person if a new topic must be introduced.
U = Unsticking:
    1. Help the person become "unstuck" when he or she uses a word incorrectly by suggesting the correct or missing word.
    2. Repeat the person's sentence using the correct or missing word.
    3. Ask, "Do you mean . . . ?"
S = Structure:
    1. Structure your questions to give the person a choice of response.
    2. Provide only two or three options at a time.
    3. Provide options that the person would like.

E = Exchange:
  1. Keep up the normal exchange of ideas we find in conversation.
  2. Begin conversations with pleasant topics.
  3. Ask easy questions that the person can answer.
  4. Give the person clues as to how to answer.
D = Direct:
  1. Keep sentences short, simple, and direct (subject—verb—object).
  2. Use and repeat nouns rather than pronouns.
  3. Use hand signals, pictures, and facial expressions.

Naomi Feil (1993) articulates an approach for caregiver communication that emphasizes discourse and enhanced quality of life of people with dementia. While the "validation breakthrough" remains to be verified through scientific method, it is suggestive. Feil, a gerontological social worker, presents anecdotal evidence on behalf of validation. She assumes that beneath the disorientation of the person with dementia there remains "a basic humanity that we all share" (1993, p. xxv). This may sound too optimistic, although Feil presents numerous episodes in which individuals affected with dementia, when "validated," manifested more residual self-identity than might be expected. Detractors may ask whether validation therapists acquiesce in a degree of subjectivity bordering on deception as more capacities are attributed to the person with dementia than are really present.

To highlight validation, it is contrasted with "reality orientation," an approach developed in the 1960s in which caregivers must constantly correct the disorientation of the affected individual. For example, "reality therapy" requires that a 90-year-old woman who remarks that she needs to visit her mother be told that she is in reality 90 and her mother is no longer living (Feil, 1993, p. 130). Proper orientation to time and place is thought to bring the affected individual back into reality. Reality therapy does have benefits when dementia is still mild; for example, it may successfully reorient the disoriented individual to circumstances as they are, or it may encourage the person with dementia to develop capacities that compensate for lost ones.

Validation therapy, on the other hand, accepts the worldview of the AD-affected individual and attempts no correction. If the individual thinks that the lamp shade is a hat, then the caregiver should not contradict this. Validating caregivers (a) enter into the world of the affected individual, serving as facilitators rather than as teachers, and (b) try to "restore well-being through nonverbal stimuli, including music, movements, and the sharing of feeling" (Feil, 1993, p. 131). This approach is useful once dementia becomes severe.

Feil claims that when AD-affected individuals are cared for in these ways, some dormant speech may reappear, negative behaviors will decrease, and the dementia will not progress as far or as fast (1993, p. 25). Anxiety and related behavioral difficulties can be ameliorated when the caregiver is an empathic listener who does not judge the disoriented person's view of reality—a view frequently rooted in the person's distant past after orientation to time is lost. Rephrasing, close eye contact, a clear and loving tone of voice, mirroring the person's motions and emotions, and touching the person on the shoulder with one's hand are all recommended aspects of validation. Feil states that even a few minutes of validation daily can be very helpful to the affected individual (although again, this is anecdotal and scientifically unverified).

Trusting and genuine relationships with many AD-affected people are possible. Caregivers have been taught to sing old, era-appropriate tunes with patients who appeared to enjoy them. For example, a 90-year-old woman with severe dementia came to life and was able to sing part of a song. Behavioral problems are reduced without the use of drugs and physical restraints. A crucial factor is the continuing belief in the potential of the person with dementia. By validating feelings through these techniques, people with dementia are able to use their remaining capacities to the maximum.

On behalf of validation, it seems to make some sense that nonadversarial and noncorrective caregiving will enhance the emotional well-being of AD-affected individuals. Consistent with Feil's concept of emotional validation is Carly R. Hellen's recommendation for activity-focused care that draws out the remaining cognitive, physical, and emotional abilities of the person with dementia (1992). According to Hellen, the person with AD should not be pressed "into a medically focused concept of caregiving" (1992, p. 1). We need a conceptual shift from illness to possibilities, from inabilities to abilities: "Residents with dementia are often more capable than either they or their caregivers realize or expect" (1992, p. 2). Caregivers should try to do less "for" or "to" and more "with." Dignity and an inner sense of worth for the affected individual are related to participation and recreation. The resident is not just "combative" or a "troublemaker," but a person. Activity-based care supports "the residents' needs for acceptance and validation as persons of worth" (Hellen, 1992, p. 50). Quality of life requires a "user friendly" environment; a positive sense of self for the affected individual is possible when caregivers facilitate emotional adjustment. The moods of people with dementia are heavily dependent on positive, nurturing care.

Like Feil, Hellen rejects reality orientation: "This method of orientation communicates a focus on 'real' information about events, time, places, and people. Residents are corrected if their 'reality' is faulty. This approach can lead to escalated anxiety and aggression because the resident often becomes embarrassed and frustrated" (1992, p. 8). Hellen describes the necessary "therapeutic fib." For example, Fred's reality is back years ago when he managed a candy store. When he approaches a staff person wanting to know about a candy shipment, the validating response is "Fred, the shipment has been sent" (p. 8). Fred then goes on his way. In this case, dementia has obviously become so severe that reasonable correction to reality is futile.

Hellen also discusses the negative emotional impact of open-ended questions. Replace "What do you want for supper?" with "Would you like chicken or fish?" Words should be supplied to AD-affected individuals from which they can choose, thereby avoiding the frustration of poor word-recollection.

Spirituality, asserts Hellen, is also important for the well-being of many AD-affected individuals: "Persons with Alzheimer's disease continue to respond to their faith and inner needs through long-remembered rituals that connect them with the present" (1992, p. 100). Prayers and hymns are still familiar in many cases, especially after several repetitions. Worship in nursing homes can create "the awareness of connectedness" (p. 100).

The above studies on caregiving all stress the importance of respecting and engaging the capacities that AD-affected individuals retain. Noncognitive forms of well-being, both relational and emotional, are vital. In a hypercognitive culture, the importance of noncognitive well-being and the continued respect due the lives of AD-affected individuals can be easily overlooked. The measure of a moral society is the extent to which those oppressed by the dominant cultural image of human fulfillment and worth are nevertheless honored. It appears that caregivers, both professional and familial, must enter into the experience of dementia, attentively enhancing emotional well-being and always remembering that quality of life is a self-fulfilling prophecy.

Toward an Ethics of Dementia Care

Enhancing well-being and making the most of what strengths are still present is central to the ethics of dementia. Understanding communication methods is important to enhance rapport and diminish anxiety. Above all, the quality of life for the person with dementia is always partly subjective and is largely a matter of emotional adjustment facilitated by interactions and environment. If we think that there can be no quality of life because of cognitive deficits, then we will probably not do the things that can enhance quality. In the process, we consign those with dementia, retardation, and a host of other brain-related conditions to neglect. This is not to suggest that at some point the quality of life should not be a factor in the limitation of life-prolonging treatments, but this topic is for a later chapter.

Nancy L. Mace and Peter V. Rabins presented an interpretive key for caregivers: "Since dementing illnesses develop slowly, they often leave intact the impaired person's ability to enjoy life and to enjoy other people. When things go badly, remind yourself that, no matter how bad the other person's memory is or how strange his behavior, he is still a unique and special human being. We can continue to love a person even after he has changed drastically, and even when we are deeply troubled by his present state" (Mace and Rabins, 1991, p. 12). This is sound counsel.

In its guidelines for care, the Alzheimer Society of Canada included this introduction: "In addition to physical needs such as the need for safety, nutrition and good health, people with Alzheimer disease have the same psychosocial needs as other individuals. They need stimulation and companionship, they need to feel secure, to feel they are unique and valued individuals, and to feel a sense of self-esteem" (1992, p. 3). People with Alzheimer disease have a human right to be treated with dignity and respect in their full heterogeneity.

Dementia is both a decline from a previous mental state and a terrible breaking off from the values of dominant culture. The moral task is always to enhance the person with AD. What cues seem to elicit memory? What music or activity seems to add to well-being? How can capacities still intact be creatively drawn out? How can modalities of touch and voice convey love to the person? Rather than think of people with dementia as out of reach because of forgetfulness, or as unworthy because of cognitive disability, the moral task is to bring them into discourse in creative ways.

Even in very advanced dementia, when communication and lucidity are largely absent, there are still communicative methods of importance. The communication we have with a newborn through emotional warmth and touch can be extended to people with AD as a standard of care. These people can be reassured that someone is with them in solidarity by the simple solicitous act of touching a shoulder. This form of care is crucially important for well-being and locates a core of humanness in self and other. Such acts are included in discourse ethics as I would extrapolate from Habermas, even though these acts are silent. One act of discourse is the extension of the hand, another is the tone of voice that reassures the person. This is the sort of basic act that makes resurrection of a sort possible (Weaver, 1986).

THREE

❧ The Challenge of Respect and Beneficence

The initial task of dementia ethics is not to analyze the many specific moral issues from genetic testing to the removal of life-sustaining technologies—the topics of subsequent chapters—but rather to secure the underpinnings of respect for those people who are affected by progressive dementia.

Sporadic AD afflicts people in their sixties and seventies. However, the number of affected individuals rises sharply to an estimated one-third of those over 85, although some studies indicate that AD may affect half of these "old-old" persons (Katzman and Saitoh, 1991). There are currently 4 million cases of AD in the United States, and 9 million are projected by the year 2040. As previously mentioned, the total cost of caring for an AD patient in northern California is approximately $47,000 per year whether the patient lives at home or in a nursing home; the total U.S. national cost for AD care is estimated at above $100 billion (Rice et al., 1993). Cost adds to the vulnerability of those who are cognitively incapacitated and therefore socially marginal.

Partly because people with dementia elicit our worst fears about how we might well end up ourselves if we become "old-old," we are reluctant to listen attentively to the voices of those with dementia to better understand the nature of their experience and their concerns. My intent in the previous chapter was to explore through narrative the experience of dementia on a descriptive level and then to explore possibilities for people with dementia to be honored even to the end stages of the illness. How can society meet the challenge of respecting and protecting people with dementia?

The Possibilities for Harm

The vulnerability of people with dementia is well documented. Elder abuse and neglect significantly affect people with dementia. Abuse, especially physical and verbal, is easier to define than is neglect. Although the latter can be obvious in some cases, it is also subject to cultural variation. Abuse and neglect are correlated with caregiver exhaustion and therefore are partly preventable by social support. Unlike infants, who are utterly dependent but small, cute, and brimming with potential, the elderly person with dementia is none of these things. In *Crime and Punishment,* Dostoyevsky's young protagonist, Raskolnikov, decides to kill an old woman because she is perceived as stupid, deaf, sick, greedy, and without metaphysical depth, while he perceives himself as superior. The contemporary problem of elder abuse is large.

People with dementia are a vulnerable population in need of special protections from those without dementia, who are capable of myriad abuses of power. There is in human nature what Nietzsche termed the "will to power," and this will on the part of the strong and rational to dominate and even harm weak and less rational people displays itself regularly. As Nietzsche wrote in 1888, combining elements of rationalism, social Darwinism, and eugenics, "The weak and ill-constituted shall perish: first principle of our philosophy, and one shall help them to do so. What is more harmful than any vice? Active sympathy for the ill-constituted and weak—Christianity" (1968, p. 116). In a statement that foreshadowed the euthanizing of people with dementia under the Nazis, Nietzsche wrote: "Pity on the whole thwarts the law of evolution, which is the law of selection. It preserves what is ripe for destruction; it defends life's disinherited and condemned; through the abundance of the ill-constituted of all kinds which it retains in life it gives life itself a gloomy and questionable aspect" (1968, p. 118). Nietzsche refers to frail elderly people, for such weakened people are anathema to the "higher type of man" (1968, p. 117).

People with dementia do not enjoy the privileged position that comes with being wiser and more experienced; they have no knowledge left to convey to their children; they no longer are intertwined with the community but rather have lost the memory of relationships; and they are therefore easily transgressed and abandoned. But even in the sorriest condition of dementia, Judeo-Christianity commands, "Honor thy father and thy mother." Honor means to esteem and show respect for and applies all the more when mental powers fade. Indifference, willfulness, and wantonness must give way to honor. Dostoyevsky's message is that the potential to abuse and even kill the elderly decrepit person is very much alive in its cage, for a sinister factor lies dormant in the heart of all. Raskolnikov was simply one in whom the wolf slipped the chain, a possibility as much or more likely now than in the past as the numbers of elderly people increase.

The veneer of respect for people with dementia is always thin, as evidenced in 1989 by four Austrian nurse's aides who killed 49 elderly demented people in long-term care institutions (Protzman, 1989, p. 1). Any society with a heritage of rationalism, individualism, and market productivity must guard against the efficient dispatching of frail elderly individuals (Post, 1990b). Between 1940 and 1945 an inconspicuous agency in Nazi Germany operated from offices in Berlin at Tiergartenstrasse 4. The "T-4 Project," begun in 1939 and concluded in 1941, was directed by the Wurzburg Professor of Psychiatry Werner Heyde. An estimated 94,000 psychiatric patients were killed, some in gas chambers, others in psychiatric hospitals and sanatoriums with overdoses of sedatives. A considerable number of those killed were demented, although the exact proportion is unknown (Muller-Hill, 1988). People with dementia were dubbed "useless eaters" who wasted precious national resources. Such an attitude was in part grounded in the eugenic theories that shaped Nazi medical policies and granted moral significance or status only to the "fit," casting aside the principle that the weak of mind and body are among us in part to strengthen our tendencies to solicitude for and tolerance of those whose lives are different. This attitude of intolerance infected the German churches, which quickly set aside the theological ethic of equal regard and conformed to brutality.

While human experimentation is clearly not the most important area in which people with dementia are being harmed, Jay Katz devoted the first chapter of his classic *Experimentation with Human Beings* (1972) to the Jewish Chronic Disease Hospital case. In July 1963 three physician researchers from Sloan Kettering injected "live cancer cells" subcutaneously into 22 chronically ill and senile patients at Brooklyn's Jewish Chronic Disease Hospital. The physicians did not inform these human guinea pigs that live cancer cells were being used and injected potentially deadly material. A number of these subjects were demented. The purpose of the experiment was to measure immune response and see if the cells would take hold and grow or would be rejected, which was more likely.

Radical Moral Equality

In our own hypercognitive culture, currently so captivated by eugenic images of human perfection both physical and mental, it is easy to think that people with dementia simply do not count morally; that is, they lack any moral significance. We divide "them" from "us," drawing a line between the rational and the less rational, the unforgetful and the most forgetful, thereby exposing people with dementia to a vulnerability manifest in disregard of their remaining capacities, subjectivity, and well-being. Abuse and neglect of people with dementia is a perennial tendency.

Sociocultural assessment of worth is notoriously exclusionary and must be rejected in favor of inclusive unconditional equality. The propensity to think more highly of some lives than others must be restrained by the principle of incomparable human worth that everyone has as a human being. For the religious ethicist, human beings are unequal in all sorts of ways but ultimately none of this overrides the fundamental equality that all people share in relation to God, making social worthiness morally irrelevant (Ramsey, 1970). However, this view need not preclude limiting the use of life-prolonging treatments for those with dementia, either by advance directive or by family consensus, another topic deferred for later analysis.

Religion at its best should provide a framework for radical equality. Judaism is a bastion of unconditional attentiveness to the frail and needy elderly individuals (Wechsler, 1993). The Psalmist wrote, "Do not cast me off in my old age, when my strength fails me and my hairs are gray, forsake me not, O God." As John Herman Randall summarized it, "The core of Hebrew morality is the conviction that in every man there dwells a holy, precious thing, never to be violated by others, expressing itself in this very refusal to violate and in respect for its fellows" (Randall, 1926, p. 42). The essential expression of steadfast active love for the vulnerable is *chesed.*

In Christian ethics, caring for the weak and outcast is a special vocation: "I was sick and you took care of me . . . just as you did it to one of the least of these who are members of my family, you did it to me" (Matt. 25:36); hospices for the frail and infirm were built from the third century. Christianity understands people with dementia as deserving of steadfast and unconditional love, or *agape,* rather than as failed rationality. There is a basic ontological equality between persons—all are equally the children of God from whom dignity and inviolability are bestowed. This encouraged the "minute and scrupulous care for human life . . . in the humblest forms" (Lecky, 1955, p. 34). Or as another historian of Western morals points out, when Christianity extolled altruism and promised heaven to the meek and "poor in spirit," it set up as virtues much that was contrary to Rome (Brinton, 1959, p. 163). Richard Tarnas summed up the Christian transformation of Western ethics as bringing about "a vital concern for every human soul, no matter what level of intelligence or culture was brought to the spiritual enterprise, and without regard to physical strength or beauty or social status" (Tarnas, 1991, p. 116).

But the most systematic and respected philosophical statement of this genealogy of morals is that of Charles Taylor, who attributed the Western moral assumption of the dignity of the most vulnerable and imperiled of body or mind to the "background picture" of Christian spirituality and theism that Nietzsche correctly identified as the historical source of the rise of the weak (Taylor, 1989).

However unacceptable is a vitalism that demands the continuation of bodily life at all costs, the Jewish and Christian notion of the sanctity of life underlies the common assumption that the most vulnerable should be protected, even if modern ethicists are insufficiently versed in the genealogy of their secularized constructs to appreciate what Taylor called "inescapable" historical frameworks. The chief virtue of this Judeo-Christian framework is that it asserts the moral status and dignity of people such as those with dementia. Their worth as human beings is assessed not in relation to social value, productivity, and rationality, but in relation to the deity, and is therefore absolute.

It is this sense of radical equality, coupled with the ideal of love (solicitous service) for even the most alien neighbor, that can embolden us to cross the boundary line of hypercognitive values in order that people with dementia not be left alone. We should not condone the existential and cultural flight from dementia that is fueled by our only partial acceptance of human realities and of our own human selves.

This revaluation of values holds out the possibility of success despite the failure of minds. We must side with the less fit and the easily forsaken. The human being is not falsified when robbed of memory and afflicted by mental powerlessness.

Well-being can certainly be partially understood in terms of cognitive abilities, including clear thinking, articulation, calculation, memory, and judgment. But our Enlightenment culture displaced the medieval and Renaissance appreciation of the "fool," so well articulated by Erasmus, with the light of pure reason. Would not the value of the person with dementia be interpreted differently in a culture that could see worth in things other than purposeful rational activity? As Michel Foucault argued, before the seventeenth century unreason was considered not a menace but a part of everyday medieval life, as "fools" walked the streets and were even considered holy recipients of a special grace liberating them from the pains of the world and from unhappiness. But unreason became a scandal and a threat in the Age of Reason, allowing a sharp segregation between "them" and "us" (Foucault, 1965).

The context for human meaningfulness and value shifted from the irrational divine drama of faith best captured in Dante's epic to the rational projects of worldly progress. Marked limitation in intellect and memory became culturally unwelcome and for this reason creates vulnerability.

A hypercognitive and secularized culture struggles to be loyal to people with dementia because it makes moral status conditional on memory and cognition. There is no more disturbing articulation of this exclusionary tendency, as emphasized in the previous chapter, than the writings of biomedical ethicists who require that human beings fulfill myriad rationalist "indicators of personhood" before they are considered of moral significance and concern. Michael Tooley, in his famous justification of infanticide, settled on the view that only if something can recall some of its past states and envisage a future for itself as well as have desires about that future, is it "intrinsically wrong to destroy it" (Tooley, 1983). Tooley's apologia for the killing of infants because they do not measure up to "personhood" could easily be applied to many people with dementia. Fortunately, most of us are not so exclusionary when it comes to loyal caring for those at the beginning and the end of life.

The "ethicists" of exclusion contribute to the negative metaphors and analogies that divert attention from the possibilities for enhanced well-being. Why act with solicitude when the self appears "gone"? Why feel anxiety over the fate of one who is, as one of my undergraduate students remarked, "only a cell culture"? Thus, people with dementia are the victims of metaphorical dehumanization and de-equalization that excessively rationalistic prerequisites for moral inclusion inevitably generate. We must reject these prerequisites.

Metaphors commonly heard in discussions of people with dementia reveal cultural values, for they capture our propensity to exclude from moral standing those who are below cognitive standards. Is the patient only a "shell" of his or her former self, a mere "husk"? Is the glass "half empty" (Howell, 1984)? Shall we think of dementia patients as "useless eaters," as "life unworthy of life?" Ethically, there is much at stake in the culture's metaphorical images of the experience of dementia, for these images will surely shape our response to this growing moral challenge (Lakoff and Johnson, 1980). Shall we nurture the well-being of people with dementia, shall we give them a disrespectful and insensitive pseudo-care, shall we efficiently dispatch them to a prompt death?

Ethics as Interpretation

Society, family members, and health care professionals *interpret* the experience of dementia, and the whole matter of moral standing and a correlative respect for persons rests on these interpretations. The dignity afforded the person with dementia is interpretive: How do we without dementia read, translate, and interpret the experience of dementia? Disagreement over the extent of our duties to demented people stems not from disagreement about the substance of an uncontroversial midlevel ethical principle such as "do no harm," but from divergent interpretations of the value of human beings who can become so forgetful as seemingly to forget who they are.

If our heuristic or interpretive key into the experience of dementia is social Darwinism and eugenics, as was the case for Nietzsche, then our sense of duty will undoubtedly diminish. If our interpretive key is a worldview that sees those who are debilitated as an opportunity for a community to manifest moral idealism, then the metaphor of "burden" will not be widely used.

We filter the phenomenon of dementia through our own lenses. No contingency of principle is involved, but "contingency of value" based on an interpretation by the observer as the experience of the dementia patient is assessed and his or her worth appraised positively or negatively (Post and Leisey, 1995). Through interpretation we picture and value the world of dementia. The observer cannot escape interpretation: scientists interpret data, literary critics provide interpretations of texts, human beings interpret one another's remarks. Interpretation is "perhaps the most basic act of human thinking; indeed, existing itself may be said to be a constant process of interpretation" (Palmer, 1969).

In interpreting dementia, it is important to avoid the tempting metaphors of shell, husk, and "gone," by which we remove people from moral significance. Such metaphors often have a powerful effect on the listener, for people tend to remember striking analogies. New analogies expose what has not been considered and uproot dogmatic mind-sets. New analogies, as much as old ones, require evaluation and must be scrutinized, for an analogy can lead to evil consequences as well as good ones. Hitler, for example, likened the Jews to vermin, an obviously hostile and outlandish analogy. But many people accepted this analogy and acted on it. The Nazis likened people with serious neurological deficits to "useless eaters," and the T-4 Project followed.

It is a mistake, however, to focus on the worst-case scenario of Nazi Germany and T-4. We too can easily interpret people with dementia in the very same negative manner. We too can think of people with dementia as "life unworthy of life," an expression that emerged in the 1920s in Germany partly in response to concerns with costs as the nation attempted to rebuild its economy after World War I. Long before T-4 and the Holocaust, in 1920, Professor A. Hoche, M.D., defined "cases of senility" as "mental death" and argued that for these people who are "inwardly unable to make a subjective claim to life," death is "no crime, no immoral act" (Hoche, 1992, pp. 259–260). Ideas and words have consequences. This view is reminiscent of the German philosopher Schopenhauer's notion that an inward "will to live" is the necessary condition for meaningful life.

We think and behave in accordance with tacit or hidden analogies and metaphors. Worldview and metaphor become intertwined and are reflections of each other. It is generally easier to scrutinize the metaphors and analogies of cultures other than our own because they leap out at us as odd. But we must equally scrutinize our own metaphors and analogies, because these define our interpretation of the world and of people with dementia.

Why Care? Ethics and Solicitude

Unduly negative interpretations of people with dementia erode solicitude, the anxiety over the good of another that undergirds all moral behavior. Solicitude, which interweaves with concepts such as care and love, depends on a positive appraisal of capacities and perceived meanings in the experience of people with dementia. The caregiver looks for some comprehensible and explanatory source of his or her solicitude: "I know that Ruth still loves me" or "Pat seems to enjoy flowers and soft music, probably more than I do." The caregiver believes that the AD-affected individual retains capacities for enjoyment and emotional warmth that are the basis or ground of solicitude. Such solicitude is property-based, that is, "When x loves y, this can be explained as the result of y's having, or x's perceiving that y has, some set S of attractive, admirable, or valuable properties; x loves y because y has S or because x perceives or believes that y has S" (Soble, 1990, p. 4).

A second form of solicitude for the person with AD is memory-based. The person with dementia may be entirely unable to remember loved ones or to communicate with them. Nevertheless, caregivers are solicitous because that person was near and dear and, no matter how dismantled, continues to be honored in reciprocation. This solicitude is still property-based, but retrospectively so. Hence one finds in many nursing homes photographs and short biographical sketches of residents with AD posted on bedroom doors by relatives for professional caregivers to see. Here the structure of solicitude is interwoven with memory, as we are reminded that "she was a wonderful and accomplished person once."

Memory-based solicitude is troubling, however, because it seems to draw some line in time between the person who was present and the remnant that is now. Steven Sabat and Rom Harre warned against the view that self-consciousness is ever gone in people with AD, because many with dementia who are presumed absent will, surprisingly, still communicate through gestures and some spoken language in the face of "quite severe deterioration" (1992, p. 459). They argued that so-called loss of self is contingent on the failure of those around a demented person to respond positively to fragile clues of selfhood. As an organizing center, the self "is not lost even in much of the end stage of the disease" (1992, p. 460).

A third and final form of solicitude is not property-based. Let us assume that in some cases there is no organizing center of the person remaining underneath the breakdown in communicative and other capacities (although I reject this assumption). As Soble put it, this view of solicitude, which is consistent with the Jewish *chesed* and the Christian *agape*, denies the need to be grounded "in y's attractive properties S or in x's belief or perception that y has S" (Soble, p. 5). Such solicitude is not property-based, nor is it explicable or easily comprehensible. Such solicitude is a matter of bestowal rather than appraisal, it is unconditional rather than conditional on certain properties in its object, and it is therefore not extinguished by unattractive properties. This solicitude "is its own reason and love is taken as a metaphysical primitive. Such is the structure of agapic personal love" (Soble, p. 6).

In the classic Western debate over the structure of love, care, and solicitude—concepts so close that I treat them as a cluster rather than attempt to distinguish them sharply—there are two traditions. Soble labeled these traditions "Plato's eros and God's agape" (p. 12). By eros, Plato chiefly meant property-based with regard to character and capacity, rather than with regard to physical beauty (he reserved the term "vulgar eros" for the latter). The common charge against the "erosic tradition" is that it lacks any security or continuity. As properties change or dissipate, the explanatory reasons for property-based solicitude diminish. The alternative is the love of bestowal that has its security and continuity in the subject. In the major study of the history of the idea of love in moral thought, these two traditions are distinguished as acquisitive and benevolent (Hazo, 1967). In modern ethics, the seminal distinction is Anders Nygren's between acquisitive love, which is determined by the "beauty or worth" of the object, and the sacrificial *agape*, which is unmotivated by worth and creates value in its object (Nygren, 1982).

Fortunately, not all solicitude is appraisive. It may be grounded in the bestowal of worth and dignity. Many caregivers will contend that the only ultimate security for people with dementia rests in a nonappraisive attitude of radical equality. Yet appraisive solicitude can be largely adequate because there is often more of a person in the person with dementia than a hypercognitive culture detects. What is morally required for dementia care is an appreciation of the noncognitive aspects of human well-being that partly rejects the Enlightenment dictum, "I think, therefore I am," and places value on the affective and social-relational aspects of being human. Nothing could be more alien to dementia ethics than pure *cogito ergo sum*. To maintain an appraisive solicitude, we must not interpret the experience of people with dementia against a background ideal of pure reason and self-control.

As James M. Gustafson noted, "I am convinced that, when we respond to a moral dilemma, the way in which we formulate the dilemma, the picture we draw of its salient features, is largely determinative of the choices we have" (1981, p. 132). What pictures shall we draw of the person with dementia? There is no ethical question more basic than this. And if the pictures are sketched with achievement-oriented, socioeconomic, and cognitive values, then harms will result.

Loss of Self?

Is it possible, in profound and terminal dementia, to speak literally of a loss of self? Does there come a point at which we can assert that the person with dementia is no longer "there," so that solicitude must no longer be property-based?

On this point I hang my argument on epistemological agnosticism. Of course, science can never verify or falsify that self-consciousness exists under any circumstances short of the complete cessation of any higher brain activity, as in the case of the persistent vegetative state—a state into which some people with dementia do enter. A vast array of neurological cases provides food for thought about the mysteries of personal identity, including issues of how essential memory really is for human identity. Perhaps recognizing the transiency of self-consciousness among normal people can erode the judgment that "the house is really empty."

Unless there is some way to disprove the existence of the self, the scientist can only be agnostic, for no patient has ever or will ever be able to express what the experience of profound dementia is like. Only if the person with dementia becomes persistently vegetative can it be said that he or she is "gone," that is, the self is clearly lost, for then there is no higher brain function even though the person is not technically dead. The most we can say about the person with advanced dementia is that there is a loss of general capacities.

The person with profound dementia must be kept comfortable and secure even if unable to communicate or act. Science cannot falsify the claim that below the breakdown in communication, an organizational center of self-consciousness lives on, and it is on this point that the reasonable burden of proof lies. No one can repudiate the interpretation that there is continuity of self underlying the progression of dementia, and it is this interpretation that bestows dignity.

In cases of profound and terminal dementia, it may be difficult to convince the observer that epistemological agnosticism is all that empiricism will permit. Solicitude is then best understood in terms of memory and bestowal. Solicitude precludes moving people with severe dementia "into the house of the dead" (Thomasma, 1989), by which I mean harm and mistreatment.

Envoi: The Caregiver as Saintly

To conclude this chapter, I invoke the concept of the saint. I am emboldened to do so in the light of what some consider to be the most important work in moral philosophy and altruism in decades, Edith Wyschogrod's monumental *Saints and Postmodernism: Revisioning Moral Philosophy* (1990). Wyschogrod wrote of an apperceptive background of daily existence in which "life is held cheap" (p. xiv). The normalization of death is "abetted by the fact that it is nightly fare on television" (p. xiv). Against this background of urban violence, wanton and unprovoked killing, and mass death, events that have defined this century as forever marred, Wyschogrod placed the saint. She did not associate the saint with any religious tradition, nor is she a neotraditionalist. Rather, she pointed out the antithesis between our death-making culture and "the saint's recognition of the primacy of the other person and the dissolution of self-interest" (p. xiv). People who are self-sacrificial and find meaning in caring for others are a striking contrast with moral decay.

To live a moral life, Wyschogrod found the narrative histories of saintly people more helpful than moral theories. The subject of hagiographic narratives is one whose adult life is "devoted to the alleviation of sorrow (the psychological suffering) and pain (the physical suffering) that afflicts persons without distinction of rank or group" (p. 34). The self is totally involved in the needs and interests of others. Wyschogrod argued for a new path in ethics that does not revert to the old but represents "an effort to develop a new altruism in an age grown cynical and hardened to catastrophe: war, genocide, the threat of worldwide ecological collapse, sporadic and unpredictable eruptions of urban violence, the use of torture, the emergence of new diseases" (p. 257).

In my conversations with family caregivers, I have found remarkable their degree of dedication and their sensitivity to the experience of dementia. Of course, not all caregivers are emotionally or physically able to do all that they would. There are limits to caregiving for the sake of the caregiver; these are explored in the next chapter on the family, which is for most people with dementia the social nexus of care.

Fittingly, this discussion concludes with an acknowledgment of the remarkable degree of caregiver self-sacrifice and solicitude for the person with dementia, which alone stands between a relatively moral civilization and the abyss of T-4. They act under and in defiance of what Wyschogrod called the "rotten sun" of our violent culture; they assert an ethic of primal trust and reliability; they do not flee from the reality of dementia that can afflict even the smoothest life with dismantlement; they understand that genuine connectedness with others entails some suffering. But how much can realistically be expected of family caregivers is a topic for the next chapter.

FOUR

❧ Familial Caregiving and the Ethics of Behavior Control

The moral role of the family is to create a framework of value and a sphere of care in which people with dementia can be found worthy of life and well-being; in addition, family caregivers must be sociopolitical advocates for affected individuals who, with waning powers of articulation and will, are politically voiceless and therefore vulnerable. Family members can challenge existing social arrangements and create within their own circle a hospitable milieu for people with this progressive disability.

The family is often uniquely solicitous because of a deeply personal memory of and gratitude toward the affected person before the onset of illness. There is among family caregivers a loyalty based on this gratitude without which "society simply could not exist" (Simmel, 1950, p. 379). All reference to gratitude aside, empirical studies have pointed out that many spouses also continue to value their mates as unique persons "despite cognitive impairment and sometimes difficult behaviors in the afflicted spouse" (Wright, 1993, p. 101). In other words, they continue to find fulfillment in the quality of their lives together, however complex the marital relationship becomes, sexually and otherwise, when someone is affected by AD (Wright, 1993). There is a familial bias toward nonappraisive solicitude and bestowed respect that professional caregivers may approximate but will rarely equal.

In the previous chapter I argued that the person with dementia is significantly disadvantaged in a society for which the image of human fulfillment is framed by cognition and productivity. An alternative framework might value creativity as much as knowledge and see worth in the lives of people with dementia, simply on the basis of their continuing capacity for creative even if irrational events (Berdyaev, 1937); another framework might value affective expression as much as knowledge and see worth in lives because of emotional interactions (Kitwood, 1993). Although it is easy to point to cases of familial abuse of people with dementia, the remarkable fact is that spouses and adult children in the U.S. remain the center of caregiving and usually provide a haven for people with dementia, in which cognition and productivity are not required.

A nine-year representative study of 1,598 urban elderly people indicated that 70.8 percent of those with cognitive impairment reside in the community and that adult children caregivers are more likely to allow for long-term continued community residence than are elderly spouses (Ford et al., 1991). In other studies, female gender and living alone predict institutionalization (Branch and Jette, 1982). Women tend to outlive men and are thus present in much higher numbers in nursing homes. The fact that so many people with dementia are cared for by their families in the community indicates that for AD-affected individuals, the family is often but not always the linchpin of solicitude. Family caregiving therefore merits significant ethical analysis.

Realistically considered, the modern nuclear family— parents and children living as an isolated unit, perhaps with grandparents in the home or nearby—faces a caregiving crisis with the rise of large numbers of people with AD. The nuclear family is the last remnant of the extended family, and public policies in support of it are far from ideal. Politics aside, the caregiving within the family is a precious moral resource—so precious that it should not be exhausted. This is why, if the family is not to be burdened beyond reason, the ethics of behavior control must be linked to a significant degree with caregiver needs as well as with the well-being of the affected individual—a linkage that frames this chapter (Light and Lebowitz, 1989). There must be some balance between what is best for the person with dementia and what is best for the caregivers (Coughlan, 1993). It is wrong for caregivers to state, "We just want to do what is in her best interests, and we have no concern about what's good for us," because the interests of the person with dementia and of his or her caregivers are practically and ethically interwoven and interdependent.

The stories of how family caregivers succeed day in and day out with people affected by AD are at least as interesting as the quandaries of death and dying or the latest living will. Success is not easy and often partial, despite the best efforts of the best caregivers. This is because of the behavioral complexity of the experience of dementia. Kenneth Solomon and Peggy Szwabo have studied the subjective experiences of people with dementia, with an interview study of 86 subjects (1992). Memory loss, disorientation, apraxias, aphasias, agnosias, increased impulsivity, sleep disturbance, diminished problem-solving skills, and exaggeration of premorbid personality are all well-known manifestations. The affective responses associated with the person's awareness of diminished intellectual and cognitive functioning are anger directed at others (58.1%), nonspecific anxiety (57%), suspiciousness (34.9%), and sadness (29.1%). Other feelings include frustration (9.3%), panic (4.7%), hopelessness (11.6%), self-blame (10.5%), worthlessness

(10.5%), and embarrassment (4.7%) (p. 297). For some subjects, the experience of dementia was benign; five reported no discomfort and had made the necessary psychological adjustments; only five subjects reported feeling subjectively confused or "mixed up" despite awareness of diminished integrative capabilities. Depression often occurs in the early stages of AD as the person grieves over lost capacities. The goals of psychotherapy are appropriate ventilation of affect and support for continued grieving (1992, p. 306). Family caregivers dealing with these affective states will inevitably find their tasks demanding if not arduous.

Family caregivers express solicitude in correcting the environmental or relational cause of a behavioral problem, in reassuring the affected person with a touch of the hand, in promoting a sense of security through preserving familiar home routines, in seeking out the causes of symptoms and carefully limiting further exposure to causative events, in not hurrying the person, in gentle reminders and humor rather than anger at forgetfulness, in attentive listening even when conversation strays, and in making use of remaining capacities through activity-focused care. All of these endeavors uphold the dignity of the person with dementia (Gwyther and Blazer, 1984).

But for those caregivers who have struggled with frightening and persistent agitation, aggressiveness, and combativeness in affected individuals, the above approaches may be insufficient. It is no easy matter to get the combative and resisting man with advanced dementia into the shower. To preserve the environment of family caregiving, restraints on such behavior are imperative, even if they serve the needs of the caregiver as well as those of the affected person.

Alistair Burns and Raymond Levy (1993) report on their 12-month study of 178 elderly patients with AD (mean age, 80.4 years; mean duration of illness, 63 months). Of these, 17 percent had experienced hallucination since the onset of illness, 16 percent were deluded (especially delusions of suspicion and theft), 20 percent had paranoid ideation not held with delusional intensity, 24 percent appeared depressed, 20 percent manifested aggressive behavior, 19 percent wandered excessively, and 48 percent experienced incontinence (1993). Medical technology, including behavioral intervention with psychotropic drugs if needed for defined purposes, certainly has a role in coming to the aid of both the AD-affected person and the caregivers.

Caregiving and Society

Caregiving obligations, capabilities, and capacities within the family are limited. Yet some caregivers have sacrificed themselves radically out of love for a family member with cognitive deficits, and paradoxically, they claim to have discovered themselves in the process. By losing themselves they find themselves. For example, one mother caring for a child with retardation described an initial sense of self-pity and overwhelming tragedy followed by acceptance, a sense that she is able to give care successfully, and finally an anger that society is not providing adequate services in support of care. This led her to political advocacy (Darling, 1979). Other caregivers may thrive from the outset because they find caring to be the most meaningful human activity, especially if they are part of a community with a narrative of nonappraisive solicitude at its core (Hauerwas, 1986). While this ethic of meaningful self-denial that is paradoxically self-discovery may not be for everyone, its perennial power must be respected, and those who live by it praised. Moreover, it is an ethic that may be more at home in ethnic minorities with a strong acceptance of human interdependence than it is in the context of Yankee independence and self-reliance (Flack and Pellegrino, 1992).

Clearly the notion that "love beareth all things" can result in oppression and harm for family caregivers, usually women, and is therefore properly suspect. Love, however, bears many things. If caregivers are denied all personal interests and serve only the interests of others rather than of self, this is patently unjust. Nevertheless, our pedagogy of the oppressed must not go so far as to ignore the remarkable depths of genuine idealism and the possibilities for fulfillment that caregiving affords when taken up with a sense of vocation.

The extent to which any given caregiver will be able to care is in part a matter of the meaning attached to such actions. Differences of meaning issue in considerable heterogeneity with regard to caregiving; for some, caregiving will be pure burden, and for others, fulfillment. For most, it will be some of both. Caregiving, like the experience of dementia itself, is interpreted through some heuristic filter that colors it, thereby adding or detracting from its meaningfulness. The evaluation of caregiving is a matter of worldview and moral narrative and can vary dramatically between communities.

Well before caregivers approach exhaustion, it is the responsibility of communities of care, whether religious or secular, to provide assistance. As was pointed out by Robert Bellah and colleagues, there is more moral idealism in American communities than we know how to articulate, despite the inroads of narcissism (Bellah, 1985). Where communities of care do not exist or are insufficient, state aid is necessary. However, the classical political philosophical principle of subsidiarity indicates that what family, religious groups, and community can accomplish by mobilizing moral commitment ought to be encouraged; one of the things that people with dementia contribute to society is a reminder that we are all ultimately interdependent. Family caregiving is too valuable to be overwhelmed.

Caregiver respite, counseling, public and private financial aid, adult day care, support groups open to caregivers and people with dementia, and visiting nurse support should all be available as needed to prevent excessive strain on caregivers. Respite services provide supervised activities appropriate for people with dementia, allowing caregivers time during the day to run errands, keep appointments, shop, or whatever. People with dementia and their caregivers are often better served by respite than by the tertiary-care hospitals with their still inadequately tempered bias—often shaped by bad laws—toward technological interference with good death (Reifler, Henry, and Sherrill, 1992).

Even with assistance, limits on familial caregiving will exist contingent on the psychological and cultural context of the caregiver. It is poor public policy to press caregivers to the point of exhaustion where they will in desperation surrender their parent, spouse, or child to an institution.

One erroneous policy position seems to ignore the needs of family caregivers: "If families would take care of the very young, the very old, the sick, the mentally ill, there would be less need for day care, hospitals, and Social Security and public resources and agencies" (Skolnick and Skolnick, 1980, p. 51). This representative statement is in part true, but it remains the case that the family is not an alternative to necessary public support. Too much public policy at present focuses on the needs of the individual whose family has relinquished care because of a lack of social and financial support. In fact, society ought not to allow families to become exhausted in the first place. Voluntary support groups such as the Alzheimer's Association can be as important as public support.

Given the frequent absence of support for caregivers, we must be tolerant of those who are unable to handle the stress of stewardship and therefore must relinquish direct care. Philosophers have argued that "ought implies can," that no person is morally obligated to do anything he or she could not have succeeded in doing, however strong the motivation. It is a maxim of moral philosophy and common sense that no one is bound to do the (practically) impossible. No person is morally reprehensible for having failed to do something that became virtually impossible, no matter how strong his or her character. Clearly it is tragic that family members who want to care cannot do so because of the old myth that the American family, like the American individual, must be self-reliant (Keniston, 1977).

In summary, families are deeply strained by caregiving demands that come with our aging society. This is not to suggest that extension of the human life span should be viewed negatively, or that with supportive policies family caregiving cannot weather these historically unprecedented demands. There have always been people who lived into old old age and became dependent on family caregivers, but never before have there been so many. Now that the extended family has all but vanished in the United States and is quickly disappearing in many other parts of the industrialized world, the network of caregivers that prevented too much of a duty from falling on any one person's shoulders is largely gone. Thus, when a caregiver in the nuclear family becomes ill or exhausted, then there may be no one to take up the slack. Additionally, many urban neighborhoods are so dangerous that families can only protect themselves rather than call for support. Yet fortunately, so many caregivers continue to give care.

Conjugal Caregiving

There is nothing easy about conjugal caregiving for people with dementia. Yet quality of life for many people with dementia is connected with a spouse who remains committed despite the illness. Lore K. Wright explores the impact of AD on the marital relationship in her lucid empirical study (1993). The presence of a spouse is one of the most important factors in preventing institutionalization, yet little is known about the marital relationship in this context. Wright interviews 30 couples in which a spouse is in the early to middle stages of AD and 17 couples in which no AD is present. All couples lived in the community. To mention just one finding, no sexual activity was reported in 63 percent of AD couples but in only 12 percent of well couples. A small percentage of affected men can become highly sexually active and disinhibited, creating significant difficulties.

Most couples expressed commitment to their marriage. Caregiver spouses "valued the mate as a unique person despite cognitive impairment and sometimes difficult behaviors in the afflicted spouse" (Wright, 1993, p. 101). The basis of their commitment did not, as might have been expected, shift to valuing marriage as an institution grounded in vows and faithfulness. Rather, caregivers retained an image of the spouse as a unique person. Spouse caregivers tend to exhibit faithfulness and gratitude, and relinquish care largely because of physical limitations.

Here is a case in point, edited from the account given me by a wife who struggled with caregiving for her husband, who eventually became quite combative:

Mrs. A. cared for her husband, Joseph, until he died of AD at age 72. The early symptoms began when he was 60. Mrs. A. reported that each evening Joseph would ask to go back to New York—not an obviously pointless request for a man from Brooklyn—and she would say they had to wait for something to arrive in the mail. She would never argue with him or say they would not return in the future. This settled Joseph down. He was a constant wanderer and especially at night would be moving about constantly. Joseph wouldn't sleep, and Mrs. A. could seldom rest. He liked to move furniture into the early morning hours. After a period he became combative and belligerent. Following an episode of violent behavior, Joseph went to the hospital and then a nursing home, where he was not allowed to stay because he was threatening to residents, patients, and staff. Three more nursing homes refused him until he was finally placed successfully.

Mrs. A. asked how Joseph, who used to be happy and outgoing, could have become combative? She could repeatedly explain things to him with a soft voice and this would calm him. But he eventually became too threatening. When placed on haloperidol, he became more argumentive and combative, she claims. On another medication he was more animated and aggressive in his wandering, once throwing rocks and stones at Mrs. A. and refusing to enter the house. In the nursing home that finally took Joseph, he was put in a geri chair and tied. He was also tied to the bed hand and foot because he just would not lie down. One nurse's aide said to Mrs. A. that when she visits her husband they are able to untie him because he seems to calm down: "He eventually didn't know my name, but he knew I was someone who took care of him." One day he asked, "Where's Marian (Mrs. A.)?" He did not remember 40 years of marriage anymore. Mrs. A. said she always got better results without yelling or getting angry at him, and that touching seemed to help. She thought that one particular aide did well at calming Joseph down and could leave him untied "because of her tone of voice and attentiveness."

Two centuries ago, when life expectancy in the United States was below forty years, the likelihood of a husband or wife caring for a spouse with dementia was small. Commitment "until death do us part" might have involved such caregiving, but usually death came before commitment was tested by dementia. Now dementia care is widespread and complicated by a gender factor. Wives tend to outlive husbands by several years and thus will do considerable caregiving in the home, while the chances are that they will, if demented, be cared for in a nursing home (Shapiro and Tate, 1985).

The direction in which conjugal stewardship points, even in difficult cases, is illustrated by the French existentialist and philosopher of solicitude, Gabriel Marcel. Marcel reacted against Jean-Paul Sartre's assumption that every human being is the enemy of the other, which interprets all human

encounters as forms of conflict. For Sartre, freedom and fidelity are op-
posed: freedom of self demands an individualism unhampered by bonds of
love and promise. Marcel preferred the ideals of mutual self-giving and
faithfulness to others; he rejected self-enclosed individualism for an authentic existence of commitment to others (Marcel, 1956). "Creative fidelity," argued Marcel, satisfies human longings for certainty and steadfast
love; it liberates persons from chaos and unpredictability. A model of conjugal fidelity, Marcel cared for his fatally ill wife over a period of years. It
was not knowledge but the creative act of caregiving that Marcel esteemed.

Anyone who speaks publicly about AD has encountered testimonies
from elderly spouses about the challenges of caregiving. Some ask if the
compassionate thing would not be the merciful killing of the affected individual. That this question emerges retrospectively enunciates the energy
and resources that caregiving requires, especially of a caregiver who is frail,
tired, and looking forward to the "golden years" or a peaceful retirement.
The plans of a lifetime must be put aside in the face of events over which
no one has control. Human contingency becomes terribly real.

As society ages, the pressure on conjugal caregiving mounts. Good husbands and wives with little sympathy for the interpretation of the ends of
marriage and family that centers on self-interest will nevertheless question
how much can be expected of them. They do not doubt that they are cus-
todians of one another and they are prepared to serve one another at considerable inconvenience. But they can give care only insofar as they are able.

I will conclude this section with another account from a spouse caregiver.

Caring for Mr. M., a 78-year-old man diagnosed five years earlier as having
probable AD, increasingly exhausted Mrs. M. in her role as a primary caregiver.
She had developed significant hypertension and had been seen in the local hospital emergency room with chest pain, diagnosed as angina, just before his admission to a nursing home. The most difficult things with which she was coping
over the year before his admission were smoking hazards (often burning holes
in furniture and carpets), nocturnal disturbance (up at night frequently and
becoming increasingly difficult to redirect to bed), wandering in the neighborhood (having been returned by police and passersby on several occasions),
and increasing difficulty with compliance to requests (refusing to bathe or take
medications). Several weeks before admission, Mr. M., while never violent,
made angry threats when asked to cooperate with care. He became increasingly agitated in the afternoons and evenings and was not sleeping at all at
night. He was intermittently frightened and talked about being on a plane.
Several times he thought his wife was trying to poison him with medications

and food. He became incontinent of urine and feces at night. Yet remarkably, in the early morning Mr. M. seemed to be much closer to his old self. Mrs. M. has spent her entire married life caring for her family. She felt severe shame and guilt at not being able to care for Mr. M. at home, and continued to be very involved in his care at the facility.

The above case raises the question of when a person with AD should be admitted to a nursing home. Especially when the caregiver is a frail elderly spouse, the health care professional must recommend admission as much for the benefit of the caregiver as for the affected person. While such judgments are inexact, they can often be made with consistency and reasonable accuracy. No conscientious caregiver should feel guilt-ridden about the decision to relinquish care based on reasonable self-concern. Much anecdotal evidence supports Wright's thesis that spouses tend to be remarkably loyal and prefer to relinquish care only at the point of physical impossibility.

Filial Morality

There is likewise nothing easy about filial caregiving for people with dementia. Here is a case in point, edited from the testimony of a woman who struggled with caregiving for her mother, who had frequent hallucinations.

My mother was born in 1920, and in 1985 she was diagnosed with dementia. Her paranoia was directed at me. She always thought I was stealing from her. Mother had arguments with some people in the mirror and would become very agitated. I chased these hallucinated people out of the house by screaming and waving cloth at them. This seemed to help. (Had this intervention not worked, then major tranquilizers would have been appropriate to reduce psychotic symptoms.) But Mother also had friends in the mirror and a little doll collection that she would show them. If we were driving in the car, I would put down the mirror above Mother's seat and she would again start talking with her friends, which seemed to keep her content. I repainted rooms in the house with much brighter colors and better light, and I put lots of mirrors all over. Mother wanders happily from mirror to mirror, talking with her mirror friends and her baby dolls. She listens several times a day to Pavarotti. She enjoys this and pretends to conduct. I bought a motor home to travel. Mother would come along. I would bring her dolls, music disks, and I put lots of mirrors around. I could even leave her in the motor home for a while, and she would be happy. The key for Mother is stimulation, safety, and security. I have help sometimes from my aunt and sister. A friend started to pick Mother up to go to day care, which has been wonderful.

Mother did eventually use some drugs to control her behavior. She got to the point where she wouldn't bathe at all. She didn't want to get undressed, and she would kick and scream and try to rip down the shower curtain. But then, once she was comfortable in the water she didn't want to get out.

Mother finally became incontinent, a useful excuse for getting her into the shower. But too many showers cause dryness of her skin. I sometimes almost have to headlock her to brush her teeth, but she forgets this right away so it's not a problem. A lot of her behavior is connected with how I treat her.

As the proportion of elderly people in Western societies grows larger, adult children are increasingly bound by obligations to chronically ill elderly parents. The human life span has been lengthened, leaving many elderly parents in a condition of dependence.

Filial duties are emphasized in the classical moral systems because it is tempting to set them aside. A century ago the British moralist Henry Sidgwick wrote that the obligation of children to parents is based on gratitude, that "truly universal intuition." That children have a moral duty to requite benefits is so clearly agreed upon, argued Sidgwick, that it is open to no dispute "except of the sweeping and abstract kind" (Sidgwick, 1981, pp. 259–260). He allowed that filial obligation might be limited in the case of a parent who has been irresponsible in fulfilling parental duties, although he hoped that this will not be the case.

But the tradition of filial morality has its critics. Philosopher Jane English asks, "What do grown children owe their parents? I will contend that the answer is 'nothing'" (English, 1979, p. 351). English granted that children may want to assist parents if a close bond of love and friendship exists, but her position places filial caretaking on the fragile basis of "spontaneous love." Another philosopher argued that all filial duties are inherently oppressive and result from religions founded on worship of the parental God. Do away with religion, he stated, and the total liberation from filial duties will follow (Slote, 1979).

In response to such theoretical analyses, I am quickly driven back to the ordinary person who attests to commitments in the sphere of filial morality, generally based on reciprocity for past parental care. Everett Hall, the philosopher of "common sense realism," wrote that our knowledge of values must "find its test in the main forms of everyday thought about everyday matters in so far as these reveal commitment in some tacit way to a view or perhaps several views about how the world is made up, about its basic dimensions" (Hall, 1961, p. 6). That people tend to take filial morality seriously, and that it is so firmly ensconced in so many varied traditions, indicates that it is not to be lightly dismissed by novel ethical theory.

By and large, then, the Western heritage of ethical ideas has underscored the importance of caring for the elderly parent, despite inconvenience, so long as parents have themselves been responsible as culturally defined. Gratitude for parental love and respect for the aging parent as a fully dignified human being are deeply inscribed in moral consciousness. But regrettably, between Sidgwick and the latter twentieth century, philosophers have had little or nothing to say about filial morality, though now the deep suspicions of English are available.

Not all of the philosophers are ready to jettison the concept of loving stewardship for the aging parent. Christina Hoff Sommers, most notably, wrote on filial morality in a manner consistent with religious tradition. Sommers warned against the consequences of the modern hostility to the moral practices and institutions "that define the traditional ties binding the members of a family or community." Before this century, she noted, "there was no question that a filial relationship defined a natural obligation" (Sommers, 1986, p. 439).

In an aging society, many adult children of elderly ill parents are faced with caretaking responsibilities of unprecedented magnitude. Given the proportions of the demographic transition to an aging society, we may well be at the crossroads between stewardship and the disregard of the aged. Despite the serious pressures of technologically expanded care, the tradition of stewardship and filial caregiving needs to be sustained. Without this tradition, moral chaos will quickly emerge.

Of course, for those whose parents have never been responsible, and whose parents have abused their children, filial love and related obligations would not be expected to hold. For example, a woman in her 50s brought her father into the ElderHealth Center for a dementia evaluation, but said she would never care for him because he had sexually molested her as a child. As a daughter, she felt she owed him nothing, although she was willing to bring him in once for diagnosis. She said to me that she brought him in not because he was her father but because he was "still a human being."

The affirmation of self-giving care should not obscure the fact that caregivers also need to be cared for. The self, if shattered by continual abnegations of personal interests, needs, and significant desires will not be able to sustain other-regarding activities for long, if at all. All people have legitimate bodily, psychological, and spiritual self-concerns that accompany their readiness to serve others.

Each of us knows people who, when confronted with the responsibilities of caring for a chronically ill child, spouse, or parent, have made tremendous sacrifices. There are reasonable limits to the caretaking responsibilities in such cases, although the particular point at which a person with dementia might be conveyed to a nursing home will vary from case to case, depending to some degree on the psychological and emotional good of the specific caregiver. The society has much to gain by assisting the family that would, if it could, continue to provide care. An unsupported caregiver can make valid appeals to integrity of self and proper self-concern, and such appeals should be heard.

It has rightly been pointed out that a crucial historical problem for women has been selflessness and self-abnegation rather than an inordinate love of self. It is not unusual for women to express the fear that the technological expansion of care will mean for them more oppressive bondage to what has commonly been termed their "experience of nothingness"—the surrendering of their individual concerns to serve the immediate needs of others to the extent that they do not have the opportunity to develop as independent persons. It is right to caution against having too much of the caretaking burden fall on women (Post, 1990a). Certainly filial love applies to men as well as women; it is clearly unjust to force an unequal burden on women.

Women are the ones typically called on to provide emotional support and assistance for those needing long-term care. Over the last few years, attention has been focused on "women in the middle," on women sandwiched between job and family responsibilities. The extension of the human life span means that "contemporary adult children provide more care and more difficult care to more parents and parents-in-law over much longer periods of time than ever has been the case before" (Brody, 1990, p. 13). Studies indicate that daughters or daughters-in-law are more than three times as likely as sons to assist an elderly caregiver with a disabled spouse, and outnumber men as the caregivers for severely disabled parents by a ratio of 4 to 1 (Brody, p. 35). Although results vary somewhat from study to study, about half of these women caregivers experience stress in the form of depression, sleeplessness, anger, and emotional exhaustion (Brody, p. 42). While women caregivers must be appreciated for all that they do, significant numbers of women are harmed by the gender expectation that they—and not men—embrace caregiving as their vocation in life. This is why traditional familial ethics is unacceptable.

What is required was described by Susan Moller Okin as "equal sharing between the sexes of family responsibilities," the "great revolution that has not happened" (Okin, 1989, p. 4). She made a persuasive case for the sharing of directly caring roles by men and women, and for an end to gendered family institutions, that is, "deeply entrenched institutionalization of sexual difference" with respect to familial and social-professional roles. It is morally unacceptable to encourage family caregiving and self-denial without strongly asserting that direct caregiving roles should fall as much in the domain of men as of women.

While the ethics of familial caregiving are deeply complicated by gender injustice, it is important to highlight that women are heterogeneous and many may find caregiving roles to be profoundly meaningful and even inspiring. Furthermore, adult sons frequently care directly for demented parents, not just indirectly through handling finances and other arrangements. Indeed, Judaism specifically enjoins the son to be personally engaged in the everyday emotional care of the feeble parent, although familial practice may not always live up to this ideal (Wechsler, 1993). Finally, caregivers should not be co-opted by a culture that seems to devalue caring. Gilbert Meilaender argued in an article entitled "I Want to Burden My Loved Ones" that caregiving responsibilities enable family members to establish a countercultural ethos of self-giving (1991). Our laissez-faire society is rooted in the Lockian myth of an individual in a state of nature before society with no essential connections to others nor any innate social sympathies. We need something like the Greek myths of care and the belief that in self-giving we achieve true fulfillment.

The Limits of Self-denial

The problem of caregivers left uncared for is a major one. With scarce support services, families providing home care also face the difficult problem of "competing obligations." The needs of one family member can, in conditions of scarcity, compete so seriously with those of another that the caretaker must relinquish some responsibility. Can there be a moral ordering of responsibilities? Would care for children take priority over care for the elderly because the young have had less opportunity to explore their potentials? If choices must be made, does one care first for one's children, then one's spouse, one's parents, and finally one's siblings? These questions are difficult and distasteful; I know of no moral theologian or philosopher who has attempted an ordering of family responsibilities. In an aging society, and in a technological culture that can prolong the lives of infants and others who not long ago would have passed away according to a more "natural" science, stewardship becomes more complicated; choices may have to be made concerning who can be cared for. I make no attempt here to develop a moral calculus or ordering of family responsibilities, and it may not be a good idea for anyone to do so. We must not be overly rigid in this area of ethics, since a great deal of individual heterogeneity in priorities and interpersonal prox-imities is inevitable. The ordering issue must nevertheless, in the light of the technological expansion of care, be considered by individual consciences.

The medicalization of modern life, the technological assault on death, the difficulty many in secular culture have in accepting human finitude and mortality, and the relative absence of a moral framework that views self-sub-ordination positively—these aspects of modernity have burdened individ-ual family caregivers and are related to the ethics of behavior control.

Familial Caregiving and the Ethics of Behavior Control

Questions of caregiver self-denial and its limits, of sustaining the envi-ronment of family caregiving without overwhelming and destroying it, all converge on the ethics of behavior control. Behavior control must be placed squarely in the context of familial care, which should be preserved so long as it remains of general benefit for the person with AD. No doubt most of the ethics of behavior control should focus on the affected person's best in-terests, but these interests are inevitably connected with those of caregivers.

Caregivers anticipate personality changes in people with dementia. At the Case Western Reserve University Alzheimer Center a study was con-ducted with family caregivers of thirty-eight people with moderate demen-tia of the Alzheimer type, ranging in age from 50 to 84 (mean 70.7) and ill an average of 5.3 years. Caregivers were asked to fill out a personality in-ventory. Affected individuals were on the whole more anxious, depressed, and psychologically vulnerable. This was coupled with decreases in assertive-ness, activity, and positive emotions, followed by warmth and excitement seeking. Some individuals were described as less open to ideas, less agree-able, and less appreciative of art and beauty, but increasingly imaginative. Certain premorbid personality traits, such as hostility, were associated with paranoid delusions (Chatterjee et al., 1992). Irritability, withdrawal, depres-sion, anxiety, fear, paranoia, suspiciousness, aggression, delusions, halluci-nations, wandering, and pacing can all "interfere with the patient's ability to live independently and maintain interpersonal relationships. Often it is the occurrence of these problems that precipitates institutionalization and family stress" (Teri and Logsdon, 1990, p. 42). Sleep disturbances are com-mon and may keep caregivers up through the night, although bright light treatment may mitigate this behavior (Satlin et al., 1992).

As much as possible, behavioral management should proceed through activities that creatively utilize remaining abilities and through relational or environmental modification. Art therapy is frequently helpful (Adamson, 1990). Focus on activities and assets can increase self-esteem (Hellen, 1992).

Music can help people with AD connect with parts of the brain that are unaffected (Zgola, 1987). Identifying the behavioral problem, gathering information about it (how, why, where, and when does it occur), identifying what happens before and after the problem, setting realistic goals and making plans, and rewarding the affected individual for achieving goals can be beneficial. For depression, encourage activity, plan pleasant activities, encourage pleasant conversation, provide a cheerful environment; for aggression, use a reassuring and gentle voice, approach the agitated person slowly and calmly, use touch gently, maintain nonthreatening postures, establish a calm environment with soft music and lighting, avoid arguing, avoid physical restraints because they elevate a person's perception of threat, and get help if in danger.

Studies indicate rage reactions in some patients with inferomedial temporal lobe lesions. Orbitofrontal lesions are associated with disinhibition (Tucker, Watson, and Heilman, 1977). While the incidence of rage reaction and disinhibition should not be exaggerated, people manifesting these are obviously difficult to care for. Aggressive behavior is a serious problem (Patel and Hope, 1993).

Wandering is a behavior that almost all caregivers must contend with at some point. It occurs in up to 26 percent of nursing home residents and up to 59 percent of community-residing people with dementia (Cohen-Mansfield et al., 1991; Teri, Larson, and Reifler, 1988). Some studies suggest that wandering may in fact be a way of coping with stress, especially in those who paced before the onset of dementia, and should therefore be encouraged (Algase, 1992). Etiologies include searching for some real or imagined object, restlessness, and anxiety. Many people with dementia will never wander, but with those who do, it can occur unexpectedly. One goal of managing wandering is to reduce caregiver burden (Morishita, 1990). Modifications in environment can assure greater safety (Chafetz, 1990). As much as possible, people with AD should be free to wander in a safe area, but not every home environment can be properly modified. Although physical restraints such as a geri chair are too restrictive, one caregiver reported tying his wife to a post in the center of the living room with a lengthy line of flexible pantyhose. He maintained that it allows sufficient movement with minimal restraint.

However, the ideal response to wandering is social and recreational activities such as music, dance, or organized ambulation (Mace and Rabins, 1991, p. 122). It is essential to ask what might have caused the wandering, for instance, a change in environment, some disturbing noise, overmedication leading to mental confusion, or some physical need. Modifications may be easily implemented. The National Alzheimer's Association now has a Safe Return program, a nationwide registry of people with AD that provides each individual with an identity bracelet or necklace.

Physical restraints result in an unnecessary immobility that itself is frequently hazardous, as when people with dementia struggle for freedom and harm themselves in the process. Medication has side effects, and to date there exists no clear drug therapy for wandering (Teri et al., 1992). If possible, caregivers should accept wandering as of benefit to the affected individual.

Family caregivers sometimes put tremendous pressure on the psychiatrist to "do something" quickly about behaviors that are offensive or frightening and cause emotional strain. Our society has come to expect prompt control of such behaviors, often through chemical means. Caregivers might already be "women-in-the-middle," so an aging parent in a delusional or agitated state is the straw that can break the camel's back. For these and other reasons, some of them economic, it is difficult to sustain the commitment to methods that are not destructive of whatever rational reflection remains for the person with dementia. Interventions that do not diminish the self-identity of affected individuals and that are physically less intrusive with respect to the brain may be costly (Dworkin, 1976).

While there can be no absolute guidelines in this area, it is clear that technological shortcuts can make people with AD passive rather than active agents to change. Society and families know that the human brain is the center of mentation, emotion, and personality and that ideally speaking, this ultimate perimeter of personhood should not be invaded except as a matter of last resort after less-invasive measures have been exhausted. But this ideal forms a dialectic with the realities of cost containment and family caregiver stress.

It is valid and beneficent to treat depression and other psychiatric ailments with drugs. But as Salzman emphasized, not all unhappiness or sense of uselessness in geriatric patients "represents true depression that requires pharmacotherapy" (1985). There are many instances in which social isolation or loss of meaning is the root of the problem, and these factors can be mitigated socially or religiously. Salzman recommended electroconvulsive therapy (ECT) only for those patients who do not respond to antidepressant treatment, whose medical condition contraindicates the use of antidepressants, or whose depression is life-threatening and/or delusional. ECT is very concerning because even mild dementia may considerably worsen immediately after it, and it is therefore indicated only for those who fail to respond to pharmacological treatments or who cannot tolerate them (Fitten et al., 1989).

Richard J. Martin and Peter J. Whitehouse argued that with regard to dementia, "behavioral interventions (i.e., making modifications in the environment) are generally preferable to medications for the treatment of most behavioral problems" (1990, p. 25). These authors pointed out that the use of medications is important in cases of depression, psychosis, anxiety, and sleep disturbances. But they urged a cautious use of psychoactive drugs, offering two basic guidelines: *(a)* treatment should be purposeful with the target symptom well defined and *(b)* "employ as few drugs as possible, start with low doses, increase dosages slowly, and monitor carefully for side effects." Polypharmacy and overmedication are particular problems in this patient population. Nancy L. Mace suggested caution in using drugs to reduce disturbed behaviors (wandering, restlessness, irritability) "at dosages that interfere with remaining cognitive function and at which side effects occur" (Mace, 1990, p. 95). She also stressed the importance of changing the physical or psychosocial environment first, before the use of drugs.

Our society is an overmedicated one in which polypharmacy harms many elderly people. There can be no replacement for solicitude and non-pharmacological approaches that enhance the affected self. In the ethics literature, two general value orientations with respect to drugs and mental health are often alluded to: pharmacological Calvinism and psychotropic hedonism. Psychiatrist Gerald Klerman originally drew this distinction. The first view is one of general distrust of all drugs, but especially those that are not clearly therapeutic. It favors verbal insights and self-determination. Psychotropic hedonists, on the other hand, see drugs as the first response to life's unpleasantries (Klerman, 1975). Those holding the first view might deal with a depressed early-onset victim of dementia through psychotherapeutic measures, if possible. Effort is made to engage the patient as an active agent of change, as reasonably cognitively intact and capable of basic insights. Drugs are only a secondary road, less valued than insight and self-determination, and not to be resorted to prematurely. By contrast, the psychotropic hedonist is more likely to resort to drugs immediately, since they are a valuable technology.

The person with dementia may eventually need medication as a last resort. There is tremendous pressure to make drugs a matter of first resort. There is the need to control patients in less than ideal surroundings and with inadequate personal care. Concern for pressures on caregivers (e.g., adult daughters or daughters-in-law) is valid to a degree. Music therapy, art therapy, and group activities may be unaccessible. It will never be possible to create a state-of-the-art dementia unit in every nursing home. Unfortunately, the pressure to use drugs for custodial rather than therapeutic reasons, so-called chemical strait-jacketing, will remain. Drug use for custodial reasons is a serious problem in long-term care facilities for the elderly, particularly in cases of understaffing or other institutional inadequacies.

Antipsychotics can lead to dry mouth and lethargy, while long-term use can lead to tardive dyskinesia; antimanic agents can lead to nausea, vomiting, and diarrhea. In home care, the possible need to control outbursts that can terrify a caregiver is predicated on the importance of keeping the care system intact, but major tranquilizers can also have negative consequences. Individuals who experience pleasant or nonbothersome delusions need not be medicated. It is important to appreciate the variable effects of disease and to understand that surprisingly small doses are often very effective.

The Expansion of Technology in Caregiving

Family caregivers should never feel uneasy about providing all the care necessary to enhance well-being while not providing purposefully life-prolonging technologies that seem to frustrate the wisdom of nature or of nature's God. The issue of the quality of life and who defines it in relation to treatment limitations will be the subject of a later chapter. While people with dementia, like people with Down syndrome, should not be discriminated against through undertreatment, this does not mean that every effort must be made to save the lives of those whose dementia is advanced. Family caregivers and AD-affected people who still are able must be willing to openly discuss the two "D" words, dementia and death, and make future plans—plans that may be relevant much sooner than expected.

Conjugal and filial caregiving was a more limited responsibility when the person with advanced dementia could not be rescued from death by antibiotics or technology. The ambiguity of penicillin, obviously an invaluable medical advance, is that pneumonia was known as the best friend of the old and senile; the ambiguity of artificial feeding is that the cessation of eating is a part of nature's wisdom in letting people with advanced dementia free. Unfortunately, the expression "playing God" has been captured by those who question the refusal and withdrawal of treatment, when in fact modern medicine is playing God by intervening aggressively with rescue technologies that seem to violate the good of those with advanced dementia.

The peril of overtreatment requires continuing communication and moral negotiation by families and physicians. No caregiver can succeed without actively generating concern in the physician with the ethical use of technology. In some cases, they may avoid the physician who is likely to overtreat the person with severe dementia. Regrettably, some caregivers desire overtreatment of those with advanced dementia. In response, conscientious physicians are raising their moral voices in arguing that certain treatments are "futile" or devoid of benefit and therefore ought not to be provided, although the precise definition of futility remains a matter of ongoing debate, and physicians must communicate to patients why they consider a treatment futile (Miles, 1991). The duties of the doctor in communicative ethics go beyond merely laying out for the patient a laundry list of treatment options, either orally or with the help of a written directive. The ethical physician must personally communicate, recommend, and carefully negotiate reasonable medical decisions with autonomous patients and their families.

The example of cardiopulmonary resuscitation (CPR) further illustrates the ethics of good communication. Too often geriatric patients or their families are provided with a paper form of some sort on which they check yes or no to CPR. But a paper form is meaningful only if it symbolizes a continual process of communication. Physicians should always inform patients and families of the probabilities of failure and success, of what "success" means, and of the extensive trauma often associated with CPR, which may include the breaking of ribs. The responsible geriatrician may ethically recommend against CPR, although the "do not resuscitate" (DNR) decision rests with patient or family. Without this level of communication we make a moral mockery of the art of medicine and of patient self-determination. Again, physicians are not required to present information to patients in a value-neutral and "unbiased" fashion, nor should they do so in many cases (Lynn, 1988).

While two decades ago the refusal and withdrawal of treatment ("passive euthanasia") was morally and legally controversial, it is now clearly established that all competent people of age have a right to refuse or have withdrawn any medical technology, including artificial nutrition and hydration, although there are clinicians and nursing homes that cannot countenance allowing patients to go without nutrition.

Issues of the refusal and withdrawal of treatment will be taken up in a later chapter. My initial point is that the technological society that according to one myth, liberates humankind from many endeavors, in fact can capture the person with advanced dementia and burden caregivers to an extreme that a more merciful nature would not countenance.

Envoi

Family caregivers suggest many things for effective care: create a safe and uncluttered environment, stick to familiar routines, avoid open-ended questions, speak slowly and clearly in simple words, avoid crowds, try not to contradict the person with dementia, speak softly and give lots of approval, give hugs, use common courtesy, and give the person as much fi and independence as possible (Coughlan, 1993). Whatever the empiric, tus of "validation breakthrough" technique, caregivers should be infor by its anecdotal emphasis on entering the world of the confused person w dementia (if he or she thinks that there are friendly people in the mirror or that the hat is a lamp, do not try to correct this according to your reality), on being nonjudgmental, and on attentive listening (Feil, 1993).

The ethics of dementia is to some extent a matter of making plans for the future with respect to treatment, and this will increasingly supply subject matter for this book. But to this point, I have focused almost entirely on solicitude and on the family as its primary locus. Without solicitude, as the eighteenth-century British moralist David Hume pointed out, we would not care in the least about the fate of others. According to Hume, the most essential aspects of the moral life lie in the social affections, the connections of solicitude without which there is little that moral reasoning can hope to accomplish. The critical ethical question is how we can weave people with dementia into the web of caring connectedness that promises to spare them the cruelty and abuse into which they have been and are easily thrown.

FIVE

❧ Fairhill Guidelines on Ethics and the Care of People with Alzheimer Disease

with Peter J. Whitehouse, M.D., Ph.D.

Between October 1993 and June 1994, the Center for Biomedical Ethics of the School of Medicine and the University Alzheimer Center of Case Western Reserve University, together with the Cleveland Chapter of the Alzheimer's Association, sponsored a community dialogue on ethical issues in dementia care. At monthly meetings, volunteer family caregivers and individuals with dementia of the Alzheimer's type identified and spoke on ethical issues in dementia care, following the chronology of the illness. An interdisciplinary and interprofessional group of individuals involved in dementia care listened attentively, raised questions, and discussed the issues with the volunteers. The group included directors of nursing (from long-term care settings, home health care agencies, and hospices), geriatricians, gerontologists, lawyers, ethicists, administrators, anthropologists, sociologists, political scientists, neurologists, psychiatrists, adult day care directors, and the leadership of the local Alzheimer's Association.

These practical guidelines represent a consensus statement for ideal care. We do not want to suggest that current circumstances always permit adherence to these guidelines or that caregivers who do not follow all our recommendations are not providing good care. We also understand that these guidelines largely presume a caring family, which does not always exist. The guidelines are named for the Fairhill Center for Aging, founded by the Benjamin Rose Institute and University Hospitals of Cleveland Health System. The Center was the site of our meetings and is a model of ongoing cooperation and collaboration across organizational and disciplinary boundaries.

I. Being Truthful: Issues in Diagnostic Disclosure

1. Physicians should sensitively inform affected individuals and their families about the diagnosis of probable Alzheimer disease (AD).

Discussion. The communication of the diagnosis should occur in a joint meeting with the affected individual and family to provide the individual with emotional support, except in rare cases when the individual objects to this. Almost without exception, individuals and their family members approach clinicians together to jointly understand the diagnosis and its implications for the future of the family unit. Hence, confidentiality is seldom a concern, but it may be.

The content, timing, and manner of disclosure must be appropriate for the affected person and family, consistent with cultural variations and values, as well as with knowledge of family dynamics. Disclosure of diagnosis should allow sufficient time for questions from family and the person diagnosed and for recommendations from the physician and health care team. It is helpful to include in the family meeting an additional member of the team, such as a social worker or nurse, to follow up on questions and discuss recommendations and resources. A follow-up session is beneficial to further discuss the diagnosis and available support systems.

As a result of the communication process, the affected person and the family should come to understand that (a) the loss of memory is not normal, but results from changes in the brain; (b) expectations for the future are uncertain, but in general, predictable; (c) while the disease cannot be cured, many of its effects can be treated; (d) support groups, such as those sponsored by the Alzheimer's Association, are available and effective; and (e) the health care team will be available to provide assistance throughout the disease process (Foley and Post, 1994).

Counseling and other services to facilitate emotional adjustment to the diagnosis are available for those who have been diagnosed and for family caregivers. Even when support is limited, disclosure is appropriate; most individuals already sense that routine functioning is diminished and are frustrated by poor recall or expression. Disclosure of diagnosis will frequently be met with the response that this is what was suspected all along. While the diagnosis of AD requires emotional adjustment that is often difficult for the affected person and family, with support it can be accepted. As cognitive function erodes, the person will eventually no longer retain information about the diagnosis nor be distressed by it; for those whose dementia is already advanced, diagnostic information may not be meaningful or warranted.

2. With diagnostic disclosure comes the responsibility to direct the affected individual and family to available resources.

Discussion. A specific care plan should be discussed and agreed upon. Nurses and social workers can be especially helpful during such discussions. Emphasis should be placed on the health care team's availability to give direct assistance or to make referrals. Although the dementia cannot be cured, the team should emphasize that efforts will be made to treat its effects and to assist the affected person and family in coping with the illness.

Telling individuals about their diagnosis allows them to plan how to most enjoy the remaining years of relatively unimpaired mental functioning; they can make medical plans, including executing advance directives (durable powers of attorney for health care or living wills), and consent to participate in AD research. Most importantly, disclosure permits the person with dementia to participate in counseling and support-group interventions, thus helping to alleviate anger, self-blame, fear, and depression (Lipkowitz, 1988; Riley, 1989).

The apolipoprotein E genetic susceptibility test for AD is a very recent development. There have now been enough studies to conclude that there is increased risk for Alzheimer disease (AD) associated with the ApoE4 gene allele and decreased risk with the E2 type. But there is *no* reliable test for increased risk, because of the statistical complexity of the data. Even without scientific validity and with no ethics guidelines in place for AD genetic testing, one pharmaceutical corporation has marketed the "ApoE GenoType Report" since 1993, emphasizing that "greater than 90% of individuals with two copies of the ApoE4 allele had late onset Alzheimer's disease, as diagnosed by postmortem pathology." Based on the research of Corder et al., (1993), the report claims to be able to indicate risk levels for all combinations of e2, e3, and e4 alleles. Susceptibility testing is ongoing at the NIA Alzheimer research centers across the United States to verify susceptibility increases, although subjects are not yet being offered test results because of the results' ambiguity (Mayeux et al., 1993).

We need ethics guidelines for genetics testing, addressing such issues as informed consent, pre- and posttest genetic counseling, the potential controversy regarding prenatal counseling, when testing should be available and to whom, and family wishes to know results of family members' tests. In view of the dementing characteristics shared by AD and Huntington disease (HD), both of which are incurable neurodegenerative diseases, it is prudent to consider predictive testing programs for AD in the light of the HD guidelines (Brandt et al., 1989; Karlinsky, Lennox, and Rossor, 1994).

II. Preserving Privileges: Issues in Driving

1. Diagnosis of AD is never itself sufficient reason for loss of driving privileges.

Discussion. An early and highly sensitive issue for many people with AD dementia is limitation of driving privileges. In many cases, the person's freedom and self-perception are threatened by limits on driving. Especially in cultural traditions that emphasize independence, autonomy, and control, relying on others for transportation can be perceived as demeaning. Moreover, driving can have tremendous significance as a symbol of individual freedom, and limitations can be an unwelcome sign of dependence.

Individuals with AD are at risk for driving impairments; if they are actually impaired, privileges must be limited for the sake of public safety (Gilley et al., 1991). Eventually all people with AD dementia must stop driving when they are a serious risk to self or others.

People with mild-to-moderate dementia present a more complicated situation. Individuals are often capable of driving for several years or more after diagnosis, depending on the rate of disease progression and on when the diagnosis is made (Hunt et al., 1993). Partial limits can be designed for the individual who may be able to drive safely in familiar surroundings, in daylight, or in good weather. Although there is an indisputable duty to prevent people from driving if they clearly threaten community safety, this principle should not be applied prematurely or without individualized risk appraisal demonstrating impairment of driving ability (Drachman, 1988).

Significantly, the most thorough recent study indicates that during the first three years after the early diagnosis of AD the risk of automobile crashes is well within the accepted range for other drivers (Drachman and Swearer, 1993). With voluntary restraints on driving (miles driven and familiar neighborhoods), along with informal termination of driving at a time decided by the person with dementia and his or her family, "the overall risk to society does not exceed a level well accepted for other groups of drivers" (Drachman and Swearer, 1993). In fact, the risk is considerably lower than that for young men between the ages of 16 and 24. After two to three years have elapsed since diagnosis, most people with dementia stop driving (Drachman and Swearer, 1993).

2. The person with dementia, if competent, should participate in any decision making regarding driving restrictions.

Discussion. Appropriate limits to driving and other activities of daily living can often be delineated and mutually agreed upon through open communication among the affected person, family, and health care professionals. Individual responses to proposed limits will vary from immediate acceptance to strong resistance. To encourage acceptance, the individual who agrees to limits should be assured that others, such as family members, will assist in providing transportation. Indeed, in discussions of limits related to dementia, family members can often avoid conflict with the affected individual by identifying and actualizing alternatives to overly risky activities.

Ideally, a privilege is never limited without offering the person ways to fill in the gaps and diminish any sense of loss. An "all-or-nothing" approach can and should be avoided. Compromise and adjustments can be successfully implemented by those who are informed and caring, especially when the person with AD dementia has insight into diminishing mental abilities and the loss of competence. The affected person should retain a sense of freedom and self-control.

The affected person should be a major participant in negotiations. The AD-affected person who lacks insight into the disease, however, is more likely to refuse to stop driving, resulting in imposed restrictions that may be resisted.

Restrictions on other daily activities (besides driving) have great significance for many people with dementia. For example, a person who may forget that a green light means proceed should avoid street crossings while out for walks alone. Cooking privileges are another example. A gradual, caring, negotiated approach to restrictions is best, protecting privileges and freedoms as much as possible while making efforts to substitute other valued activities for the ones that are lost. The lives of people with dementia should be as free and fulfilling as possible. A totally safe, risk-free existence is neither possible nor beneficial.

3. Whether the physician or other health professionals should have a role in the restriction of driving privileges remains unclear; such a role is highly paternalistic and is probably better left to family and community.

Discussion. Mandatory physician reporting of those diagnosed with AD singles out people with dementia and violates their right to confidentiality (Reuben, Silliman, and Traines, 1988). California mandates physician reporting of people with AD, and this information is forwarded to the Department of Motor Vehicles. The person is then required to be assessed for driving abilities (State of California, 1987). This approach frees physicians and families from fear of lawsuits (should the patient have an accident) and the need to make risk assessment, while clarifying responsibility to the wider public. However, there is no consensus that physicians should be responsible for preventing dangerous driving, since such a duty does an injustice to people with dementia by violating their medical confidentiality. Moreover, reporting may dissuade people with dementia from seeking help.

Mechanisms for referral of people with dementia by family members or the community for nonadversarial driving tests are necessary (Drachman and Swearer, 1993). Debate continues about the best methods and criteria for assessing competence to drive and about retesting intervals. Based on their observations and experiences, family members can make informed assessments of driving skills. However, a "behind-the-wheel" driving test by an examiner with special training to detect judgment problems associated with dementia may be useful in negotiation because it has the benefit of establishing a more objective assessment.

III. Respecting Choice: Issues in Competency and Autonomy

1. People with dementia should be allowed to exercise whatever competencies (capacities) for specific tasks and choices they retain, for denying this challenges their independence and dignity.

Discussion. Competent people have a moral and legal right to reject any medical treatment. Many people with less severe dementia retain this right, and it should be protected. Many people with dementia find it distressing to have their wishes overridden in areas in which they are still competent, and this should be avoided. False accusations of incompetence can leave an elderly person feeling worthless and hopeless. Even when a person is incompetent in some specific area, caregivers should seek the least restrictive alternative.

Just as it is obligatory to protect a person with dementia from seriously harmful consequences, it is also obligatory to respect his or her competent decisions. Law does not allow interference with a competent person's choices on purely paternalistic grounds. Diagnosis of AD alone is not an indication of incompetency. A person with AD may lack capacities to drive, handle financial affairs, or live independently in the community, but still have the capacities to make competent decisions about place of residence and medical care.

Judgments of incompetency should reflect the mental condition of the person with dementia, not the needs or intolerance of others. Individuals may be unwelcome in the community because they are remiss about hygiene, uninhibited, inclined to mishaps, and unable to keep their residences in good appearance. Appointment of a legal guardian for specific tasks (e.g., financial affairs) might allow them to remain in the community and maintain a degree of independence (perhaps with help regarding cleaning, etc.). In cases of potential relocation, it should be remembered that the beneficial processes of life review and reminiscence are associated with residing in a familiar and meaningful place (Post, 1993b). Thus, relocation can itself result in harm to the affected person (Spar and LaRue, 1990, p. 21).

Concern for the autonomy of people with dementia requires that competencies or capacities be assessed for specific tasks ("functional assessment"). The locus of power to make decisions rests on this assessment, so it should not be made lightly. Rather than a single ability that people possess or lack, competency is composed of a series of abilities, some of which may be present while others are absent.

Conflict arises when the person with dementia insists on doing something that he or she is incompetent to do, failing to recognize intolerable risks to self or others. In such cases, legal guardianship may be necessary. For example, a person with dementia who insists on a particular style of cooking despite having caused one or more fires in the apartment may require a guardian with the power to determine circumstances or even place of residence. Guardianship is an extreme measure, however, which can usually be avoided with good communication and creative intervention. While good care requires an acceptable level of safety, risks should not be exaggerated.

2. In almost all cases, judgments of competency in health care settings for medical decision making can be made without the need for legal proceedings.

Discussion. In medical contexts, rough judgments of specific competency are routinely made informally by attending physicians, other health care professionals, and family members. Competency assessment can be straightforward and based on common sense, for example, when an elderly patient is obviously incoherent in conversation, retains little or no information, responds to the same repeated question with seemingly antithetical statements, and lacks insight into the consequences of a decision or its alternatives. Information is neither grasped nor manipulated. There is no validity to protecting an autonomy that the person does not possess.

Yet this same person may be obviously incompetent one day but competent the next. Even the person with somewhat advanced dementia may have intermittent periods of lucidity that allow significant decision making. Some are relatively lucid in the early hours of the day but grow less so as they tire.

A person with AD may have scored badly on the Mini-Mental State Examination or some other test of cognitive impairment. For people who are marginally competent, however, these tests do not determine task-specific ability. Questioning and discussion are necessary to examine understanding and reasoning capacities for the specific task at hand.

Most assessments of competency in the health care setting are made informally by the primary care or primary attending physician (Appelbaum and Grisso, 1988). Knowledge about the person with dementia and his or her values can be important in determining competency, because decisions consistent with long-held values are more likely to be authentic. Primary care physicians are able to make sound judgments about competency. When such judgments are difficult, the attending physician may request a formal psychiatric evaluation.

Competency, whether clinical or nonclinical, includes the ability to understand the relevant options and their consequences in the light of one's own values. The standard definition of competency for medical treatment decision making includes the essential element of the patient's ability to understand the nature, purpose, risks, benefits, and alternatives of the proposed treatment. More specifically, a patient needs to be able *(a)* to appreciate that he or she has a choice; *(b)* to understand the medical situation and prognosis, the nature of the recommended care, the risks and benefits of each alternative, and the likely consequences; and *(c)* to maintain sufficient decisional stability over time, in contrast to the profound vacillation that indicates an absence of capacity (Lo, 1990). Reasonable indecision or change of mind does not in and of itself indicate incapacity. During routine conversations, however, a person with advanced AD can vacillate from one moment to the next in complete self-contradiction, a clear indication of incompetency.

Judgments of competency with respect to property are usually made while the patient is living in the community; in the absence of a power of attorney, such decisions require legal action to establish property guardianship. In the clinical context, courts and legally appointed guardians are rarely involved in judgments of incapacity to make treatment decisions. Judgments of competency for health care decisions can be made informally, avoiding legal entanglement.

Competency assessment requires a "sliding scale" (Buchanan and Brock, 1990). If a patient refuses a clearly beneficial surgery that promises to restore a better quality of life, a relatively high standard of competence and measure of certitude would be desired before honoring such a request. If the consequences of a decision are minor, the standards of competence can be lower. Only the law can declare incompetency in medical decision making, thereby overriding treatment refusal.

3. It is important to plan for the global incompetency of advanced dementia through the use of living wills and other advance directives.

Discussion. Estate wills, living wills, and durable powers of attorney for health care are necessary to extend one's competency and autonomy prospectively after diagnosis of probable AD. The precedent self that is fully intact prior to the clinical manifestation of dementia has the legal right and authority to dictate levels of medical care for the severely demented self. It is possible to raise questions about the capacity of the precedent self to make these decisions, since he or she has not experienced the demented state and may view it too negatively; however, legally the right to determine treatment limitations is established by advance directive legislation.

IV. Valuing Freedom: Issues in Behavior Control

1. The best approach to problem behaviors relies on social and environmental modifications and creative activities, thereby preserving independence and self-esteem.

Discussion. Activities that creatively draw on remaining abilities, coupled with relational or environmental modification, can positively influence the behavior of people with dementia. For example, art and music programs can be helpful (Zgola, 1987). In cases of agitated behavior, health professionals and family members should use a reassuring and gentle voice, always approaching the agitated person slowly and calmly, using gentle touch, maintaining nonthreatening postures, establishing a calm environment with soft music and lighting, and avoiding argument (Gwyther and Blazer, 1984; Mace, 1990).

Wandering occurs in up to 26 percent of nursing home residents and up to 59 percent of community-residing people with dementia (Cohen-Mansfield et al., 1991). Some studies suggest that wandering should be encouraged as a person's way of coping with stress, especially for those who, prior to the onset of AD, responded to stress by engaging in physical activity such as pacing (Algase, 1992). Etiologies of wandering include searching for some real or imagined object, restlessness, and anxiety. Many people with dementia will never wander; for those who do, however, it can occur unexpectedly. Modifications in environment can assure greater safety (Chafetz, 1990). As much as possible, people with AD should be free to wander in safe areas. Involuntary restraint is unethical and illegal.

Because of various side effects, there is no current drug therapy for wandering that may not interfere with other valued activities (Teri et al., 1992). Therefore, if possible, caregivers should view wandering as beneficial to the affected individual and look for creative ways to allow it to occur in a safe, protective environment.

2. Physical and chemical restraints should not be substituted for social, environmental, and activity modifications.

Discussion. Physical restraints result in unnecessary immobility and are frequently hazardous—for example, when people with dementia struggle for freedom and harm themselves in the process. Strangulation, medical ailments caused by immobility, and increased agitation are among the serious and substantial harms caused by physical restraints (Johnson, 1990). Concern for the safety of the person with dementia is significant, especially because falls in the frail elderly can be very serious. But the potential harms of physical restraints must also be counted as risks to safety (Evans and Strumpf, 1989). Moreover, physical restraints elevate the AD-affected person's perception of threat (Patel and Hope, 1993). Their use is partly the result of fear of law suits against nursing homes, although such suits are rare (Johnson, 1990). While the value of safety is important, it does not justify involuntary restraint and the indignation and indignity of being tied down.

Health professionals need to be attentive to how family caregivers control behavior. Professionals may discover individualized and diverse ways of controlling behavior without resorting to chemical and physical restraints (Reifler, Henry, and Sherrill, 1992). Professionals should encourage diverse approaches by family caregivers (Teri et al., 1992).

Family caregivers may pressure physicians to "do something" quickly about behaviors that are offensive or frightening and cause emotional stress in the family. Society has come to expect prompt control of such behaviors, often through chemical means. Caregivers may already be "women-in-the-middle" dealing with various competing obligations. An aging parent in a delusional or agitated state is "the last straw." For these and other reasons, some of them economic, it can be difficult for family members to sustain the commitment to environmental and psychosocial methods (Dworkin, 1976). In such circumstances, families may need to rely on pharmacology to a greater extent than they might otherwise. If competent to do so, however, people with AD may refuse medications.

3. Behavior-controlling drugs should be used cautiously and only for specified purposes.

Discussion. With regard to AD, environmental interventions are often preferable to medications for the treatment of most behavioral problems. Medications can be appropriate for treating depression, psychosis, anxiety, and sleep disturbances. If psychoactive drugs are used, the purpose of treatment and the target symptom must be well defined; as few drugs as possible should be used, starting with low doses, increasing dosages slowly, and monitoring carefully for side effects (Martin and Whitehouse, 1990).

Polypharmacy and overmedication are particular problems in the demented patient population. Drugs to reduce disturbed behaviors (e.g., wandering, restlessness, irritability) create ethical issues when used at doses that interfere with remaining cognitive function and cause other side effects. Clinical experience and scientific evidence indicate that patients' behavior can be controlled at lower dosages than are commonly given. Ideally, efforts to change the physical or psychosocial environment should be tried before drugs are prescribed.

Most families want to keep the person with dementia at home if possible (Ford et al., 1991). Used sparingly, drugs can have desired therapeutic effects, maintain the home care environment, lighten the burden on caregivers, and make the use of physical restraints unnecessary. Thus, when used carefully to attain defined short-term goals, drugs can be highly beneficial (Light and Lebowitz, 1989). They can make caregiving more manageable without compromising the person's quality of life.

It is important to recognize the reality of caregiver limits in a family setting. It is not to the advantage of the person with AD to remain in the family setting if caregivers either do not wish to provide care or are unable to manage the situation. Public policy often does not provide enough community support. There is no shame in resorting to facility-based care if necessary.

4. An individual profile of the person with dementia should be available to facility-based caregivers (nursing homes, assisted living, or other care settings), highlighting an interactive and activity-based care plan known to be most effective for the individual.

Discussion. As an admission policy for nursing homes, an interview with family caregivers and interaction with the AD-affected person should determine which environmental, social, and activity-based interventions are helpful for the particular individual. The reportedly effective interventions should be noted in the individual's medical record and conveyed to the health care team. Moreover, professional caregivers can themselves learn from understanding what works for particular individuals; these discoveries should also be recorded in the individual's medical record. While nursing assistant rotation is not ideal, loss of continuity of care can be ameliorated by maintaining a written profile of the person. Nursing assistants can learn a great deal about promoting the well-being of individuals with dementia and should record this information for others.

Family caregivers need to examine the philosophy of nursing homes, matching their knowledge of the person with dementia with the profile of the institution. Family members have an obligation and right to discuss the institution's philosophy of care prior to admission. They should insist on clear goals for medications. An educated partnership is essential for promoting the well-being of the patient.

V. The Right to Die: Issues in Death and Dying

1. AD should be acknowledged as a terminal illness, thereby removing doubt about the right of affected people to refuse treatment by advance directive should they become incompetent to make medical decisions.

Discussion. AD will result in the affected person's death, usually from pneumonia. It is, therefore, a terminal condition in the broadest sense of the term—although it does not fit the narrow definition of terminal as meaning having an expected life span of less than six months. The time between diagnosis of AD and death varies, with an average period of five to seven years. Even if death is not imminent, AD is terminal. Typically, however, death is not discussed sufficiently. A good death requires that the values of the person be integrated into the process of dying.

The philosophy of hospice is very appropriate for the care of people with advanced dementia. One difficulty that should be addressed by policymakers is the Medicare requirement that hospice eligibility be determined by physician certification that death will likely occur within six months. Hospices would need to be prepared for the problems of dementia and for potentially more extended periods of care.

2. Family members, AD-affected people, and health care professionals should sensitively discuss and plan for a good death, supported by appropriate documentation.

Discussion. Family members and health care professionals may resist raising issues of values and dying with AD-affected individuals. Unfortunately, hesitancy to disclose the diagnosis of dementia and reluctance to discuss death result in many AD-affected people being denied the opportunity to make plans while they are still able.

The physician who provides continuing care for the person with dementia should initiate discussion with patients and families regarding the extent to which aggressive measures should be used to sustain life. People with mild dementia should be asked about their wishes regarding end-of-life choices. They can often respond competently.

People with dementia and their families should take responsibility for controlling the use of technologies, directing discussion toward desired goals. Many individuals prefer to limit the use of artificial feeding, mechanical ventilators, cardiopulmonary resuscitation, and other invasive technologies. The use of living wills and durable powers for health care is legally recognized by state statute, although documentation and specifications can vary from state to state. However, documents may be ignored by medical staff, requiring family vigilance to assure their implementation.

Conflicts and disagreements between affected individuals and families can best be avoided or resolved through early and continuing communication. When they are competent, many older people are clear and consistent in their views, often wanting to avoid life-prolonging technology that is not clearly beneficial. Based on the moral principle of respect for the autonomy or self-determination of the adult, family members are obliged to honor the wishes of their loved ones. Health care professionals must spend time with families clarifying the importance of this respect in the medical context.

It has been argued that primary care physicians should be required to discuss values and dying with all elderly patients on a regular basis (Thomasma, 1991). Preferences regarding life-prolonging treatment can then be expressed before the development of dementia or any other major illness. This way, people with AD will not have questions raised about their prior competency by those who cannot accept the fact that the affected individual is averse to life prolongation. Health care professionals should be proactive, sensitively leading elderly people into responsible conversation and planning for the future.

3. Many people with families want to entrust treatment decisions to loved ones who will act in their best interests; this should be supported.

Discussion. Not every person with AD has trusted family members, but many do. While it is vital that physicians communicate directly with competent elderly individuals to discern and respect patient wishes, families should be part of the process of communication whenever possible. If a given cultural tradition describes personhood as essentially social and familial—that is, not belonging to itself but rather to others in relationship, then it is reasonable and ethical for AD-affected people to defer decisions to trusted others. There is evidence that some people want family members to override their documented wishes, if doing so is clearly in their best interests (Sehgal et al., 1992). Therefore, people with AD should be asked how strictly they want their advance directives to be followed.

One way to empower individual choice, while allowing family members to deal with unforeseen situations, is through an advance directive that combines the living will with the durable power of attorney for the person receiving health care. Usually, the designated surrogate who holds "the power of attorney for health care" is a trusted family member. These combined documents include a statement of values from the affected person to provide general guidance to the surrogate; they also allow the surrogate freedom to make specific decisions on the basis of substituted judgment—that is, "a good-faith effort to make the treatment decision in the manner in which the patient himself would have made it if competent, provided there is sufficient evidence on which to base such a determination" (Annas and Glantz, 1986, p. 105). This solves the problem of vagueness and unanticipated circumstances that limit the living will. Too few people prepare such documents.

It is imperative that courts not remove decision-making authority from families, in conversation with physicians, when no clear planning or documentation has been completed for an incompetent person with AD. In the Mary O'Connor case the highest New York State court ruled that, based on its perception of her wishes and best interests, a 77-year-old woman with multi-infarct dementia must be given life-prolonging treatments despite the desires of the family to the contrary. The court cited a state interest in preserving the lives of incompetent people and the absence of "unequivocal" evidence from the affected woman. Fortunately, this is an isolated case. However, such court rulings threaten the authority of families to interpret their loved ones' values and best interests (Lo, 1990; O'Connor, 1988).

People with AD, while competent, have a clear right to decide against any and all treatments and to extend that right into the future as the disease worsens and their mental abilities wane. An exception to this principle involves treatments obviously necessary for comfort and palliation, such as treatment of a painful urinary tract infection.

4. Patient refusals of life-support and its withdrawal are distinguishable from voluntary euthanasia and assisted suicide.

Discussion. Health care professionals and family members should not equate the right to refuse or withdraw treatments with assisted suicide or euthanasia (mercy killing). When a competent individual has requested not to be resuscitated ("do not resuscitate" or "DNR" orders) and his or her request is violated, society loses faith in the health care system. When people begin to fear that their right to refuse treatment will not be respected, they may view suicide, assisted suicide, or euthanasia as their only alternatives.

It is morally correct for physicians to follow a living will, even when a relative disagrees. For treatment withdrawals that are on the legal cutting edge, however, such as removal of artificial nutrition and hydration, familial consensus is desirable. Clinical ethics consultation or ethics committees may be used to facilitate consensus. Courts should be used only as a last resort for unresolved conflicts.

VI. Quality of Life: Issues in the Cultural Perception of Dementia

1. "Quality of life" in people with dementia is difficult to assess because it includes a subjective element; therefore, those who are cognitively intact must avoid simplistic assertions.

Discussion. The concept of quality of life is complex because it incorporates objective (external observations) and subjective (internal self-perceptions) elements (Birren and Dieckmann, 1991; Walter and Shannon, 1990). It is true that some of the elements of quality of life include capacities: to make judgments and solve problems; to remember recent events; to remember past events; to handle business, financial and/or social affairs; to pursue hobbies and interests; to form and maintain relationships with others; to recognize close family members or friends; to experience emotions; to recognize oneself; to plan for the future; to eat; to control bladder and bowel; and to communicate through speech. The fact that all or some of these capacities may be lost to severe dementia explains why people fear Alzheimer disease so much.

Yet, as one family caregiver in our community dialogue stated, most of us assess quality of life in AD-affected persons more negatively than is justified, largely because we hold cognitive skills in such high regard. "People of intellectual capacities would not appreciate Dad's moments of joy," she added, "but Dad really enjoyed the social interaction in the nursing home. We intellectuals are not a jury of Dad's peers."

Caregivers emphasize that what counts morally is the AD-affected person's sense of quality of life, and caregivers must respond at the affected person's level. Caregivers need to learn what makes affected people feel happy, although diminished emotional life can be another qualitative aspect of AD. An inclination toward negative judgments can lead to a failure to invest the personal and social resources that will enhance quality for the affected individual. Quality of life is partly contingent on the creation of a supportive environment to enhance the affected person's well-being.

Because a reliable quantitative measure of a patient's internal experience is impossible, quality of life has a subjective aspect that no outward observer can assess. Therefore, caution is in order. Quality-of-life judgments might be misused to rid society of unproductive members. In clinical discussions with patients or their surrogates regarding treatment limitation, reference to quality of life is not uncommon.

2. While we must be cautious about assessing quality of life, there may come a point in the progression of dementia at which quality of life is so severely compromised that many would justifiably wish to limit life-extending treatment.

Discussion. Because the severity of progressive dementia must be measured on a continuum, people may define morally significant thresholds, such as when the patient becomes mute and lacks all interactive capacities or no longer recognizes loved ones. With respect to moral significance, there will not be universal agreement on these thresholds. Some family members will state that the patient is "no longer there." Once these points have been reached, the meaning and substance of human life has deteriorated; the decision not to use medical technologies (except for comfort care) is then acceptable, though not mandatory.

Certainly in very advanced and terminal dementia (mute, bedridden, incontinent of bladder and bowel, unmeasurable intellectual functions, death inevitable), comfort care is all that medicine should offer. Comfort care means palliation only—that is, it excludes artificial nutrition and hydration, dialysis, and all other medical interventions unless necessary for the control of pain and discomfort. While some treatments (for example, antibiotics) are intended for comfort care, they may extend life as an unintended side effect, with doubtful palliative effects.

Some people believe that the long-term goal of dementia care should be comfort and emotional well-being rather than life-prolongation. If this is the established goal, it is easier to make many specific decisions about medical treatments. Quality of life should be maintained. Caregivers must continue to observe the affected individual carefully and provide whatever forms of pleasure and comfort are possible. A feeding tube will rarely be a source of comfort care; a gentle touch of the hand will. Relationships are more comforting to the affected individual than the sight of an object protruding from the abdomen.

Although more research is necessary, preliminary data (a study of forty-four alert, elderly, nursing home residents by case vignettes) indicate that a considerable majority of elderly nursing home residents would want only comfort care and palliation in the event of advanced AD; a minority desire aggressive life-extending treatments (Michelson et al., 1991).

3. Quality of life in nursing homes requires commitment to resident autonomy and respect for treatment refusals; governmental regulations should strongly uphold both of these goals.

Discussion. Since the 1950s, nursing homes have become increasingly medicalized, and residents have assumed the classic passive sick role (Lidz, Fischer, and Arnold, 1992, p. 31). In 1987, the U.S. Congress mandated new nursing home regulations focused primarily on safety and health, although the Omnibus Budget Reconciliation Act also includes training in residents' rights. As one expert states, "Nursing home regulations emphasize safety above all" (Kane, 1990, p. 17). The Institute of Medicine issued a major report emphasizing quality of life in nursing homes, based on respect for residents, as an alternative to the medical model (1986). The U.S. Department of Health and Human Services Advisory Panel on Alzheimer's Disease states clearly: "Emphasize quality of life, broadly defined, over mere survival" (Advisory Panel, 1991, p. 42).

Many nursing home professionals adhere to this principle, or would adhere to it if they could. State regulations, however, at least as they are interpreted by some state inspectors, diminish respect for resident values and treatment decision making. While regulations serve a positive protective function in many situations, they do not take into account the condition of dementia and the complexity of ethical choices that affected individuals and families must make.

Regulations concerning caloric intake provide a good illustration. Some nursing homes are fearful of allowing a person with profound and terminal dementia to die peacefully, as they have throughout the course of history. Instead, they routinely provide artificial feeding to avoid possible penalties imposed by the state when residents lose weight. It is not unusual for a nursing home to transfer a resident to a tertiary care hospital to implement a plan for withdrawal of artificial nutrition and hydration, a practice that is legally acceptable if requested by the affected individual prospectively. The transfer, however, can be a traumatic experience for the family and the nursing staff.

Even though nursing homes may run some risk of legal liability when they appropriately allow a person with advanced dementia to die, they should nevertheless do what is right and challenge the state if need be. Clinical evidence is mounting that foregoing fluids and nutrition in end-stage illness does not cause suffering; providing nutrition artificially frequently causes unpleasant side effects, such as bloating or aspiration pneumonia (Sullivan, 1993).

In some cases, state inspectors are more interested in measuring weight than in taking dementia and ethics into account. Nursing homes must insist that inspectors be better educated in ethics and that regulations be clear about the distinctive issues surrounding people with AD.

Nursing homes should involve residents, including AD-affected residents (an estimated 50 percent of residents) who are still capable, in discussions of treatment plans and must respect advance directives. When a resident progresses to advanced dementia, the capacity for goal-oriented behavior is largely absent, and the value of autonomy becomes less relevant. Two ethical principles are then paramount: *(a)* respect for the dignity of all human beings and *(b)* respect for the values and wishes of the resident as expressed while he or she was competent. Even in cases of advanced dementia, the nursing home staff must be as responsive to the resident's emotional needs as they are to bodily needs.

Nursing home ethics committees should be established to advise on specific cases involving dementia, to educate their staff and other professionals in current health care ethics, and to develop clear policies in areas such as DNR, use of artificial feeding, advance directives, and medical futility. In addition, these committees should regularly review the implementation of approved policies.

In conclusion, while these guidelines do not cover every issue that arises in the progression of irreversible dementia, they indicate the range of ethical concerns that must be seriously considered as society ages and dementia of the Alzheimer type becomes ever more frequent. As the millennium draws to a close, it is the decline of the mind contained within the still viable body that raises some of the most urgent concerns for medical ethics and society.

Acknowledgments

These guidelines were developed for the Cleveland Community Dialogue on Ethics and the Progression of Dementia, codirected by Stephen G. Post, Ph.D. (Project Director); Peter J. Whitehouse, Ph.D., M.D.; Sharen K. Eckert, Executive Director of the Alzheimer's Association Cleveland Chapter; and Ruth B. Fiordalis, President of the Board of Trustees of Fairhill Center for Aging and Vice-President of Clinical Health Laboratories, Inc. (Project CoDirectors).

Grateful acknowledgment is made of the contributions of the following members of the community dialogue: Georgia J. Anetzberger, Ph.D., Robert H. Binstock, Ph.D., Dianne Brescia, M.A., Maxine Bryant, R.N., Barbara Carter, R.N., Anne J. Chance, B.S.N, Dolores L. Christie, Ph.D., Richard E. Christie, M.D., Rebecca Dresser, J.D., Richard H. Fortinsky,

Ph.D., Atwood D. Gaines, Ph.D., Peter J. Greco, M.D., Marie Haug, Ph.D., Mary A. Kaufmann, R.N., Doreen Kearney, R.N., Betty Kemper, R.N., Alice J. Kethley, Ph.D., Judith K. Klug, R.N., Margaret Kuechle, R.N., Carolyn L. Lehman, R.N., M.S.N, Linda Lessin, R.N., Mary-Jo Maish, R.N., M.S.N, Kathleen Meyer, R.N., Thomas H. Murray, Ph.D., Elizabeth O'Toole, M.D., Laurence M. Petty, M.D., Arlene A. Rak, R.N., Julia Hannum Rose, Ph.D., Joan S. Scharf, M.S.W., L.I.S.W., Ashwini Sehgal, M.D., Margaret L. Serenari, R.N.C, Jacquilyn Slomka, R.N., Ph.D., Martin L. Smith, S.T.D, Kathleen A. Smyth, Ph.D., Nancy A. Strick, R.N., Mary Lou Strickland, R.N., M.S.N, M.B.A, Ruth E. Toth, R.N., Nancy Wadsworth, M.S.S.A, R.N., L.I.S.W., Aloise Weiker, R.N., B.S.N, Stuart J. Youngner, M.D., and Carol A. Zadorozny, N.D.

We also wish to thank Mr. Edward F. Truschke, President of the National Alzheimer's Association, for attending the final meeting of the dialogue.

We would like to thank the Cleveland Foundation, the Ohio Humanities Council, and Clinical Health Laboratories, Inc., for their generous funding of this community dialogue.

SIX

❧ Presymptomatic Testing:
An Amniocentesis for Elderly Persons

Ours is a time when uncertainty has diminished before the power of presymptomatic and prenatal testing. The elderly person who misplaces things around the house or sometimes forgets where the car is parked may worry that such events, while common in all age groups, portend descent into the world of dementia. Instead of living with uncertainty and a consequent lack of power to control and plan the future, there are many who wish to know in advance all that can be known. They look toward a test to predict dementia, and biomedical science is trying to provide one. In addition to setting one's affairs in order and getting the most quality out of remaining years that are free from dementia, there is the hope that some preventive medicines or techniques might be available. Nonvalidated recommendations abound, for example, *Life* ran a cover story in 1994 on researchers suggesting that using new areas of the brain and exercising those areas already in use can prevent dementia (read more, play chess, and take up a musical instrument). A reliable predictive test would surely send Cognex sales flying.

David Masur, a neuropsychologist, claims that a combination of four memory tests can indicate a very low likelihood of Alzheimer disease within four years of testing. The subject matches symbols with numbers, attempts to remember the object placed in a bag, tries to recall twelve words spoken by the examiner, and names objects in a particular category as quickly as possible. Masur states that he can identify a subgroup of elderly people with 85 percent probability of manifesting AD within four years, a subgroup with a 95 percent probability of remaining AD-free for four years, and a group in the grey zone of uncertainty. The study involved 317 healthy elderly people aged 75 to 85 followed for four years. Of 212 who scored well, 202 did not develop AD; of 13 with very low scores, 11 did develop AD (Masur et al., 1994). Masur contends, in essence, that he can detect AD in its preclinical stage. He believes that predictive testing will become important if preventive treatments emerge, but even now as his phones ring with requests for the test, he sees benefits—those who score well will be reassured and those who score very badly will be alerted to this fact, possibly facilitating their emotional adjustment (cited in *U.S. News & World Report,*

12 September 1994, p. 91). Some, but not all dementia specialists are critical of the Masur study.

What benefits does such a test, if confirmed, offer? At considerable expense, many in our aging population can breathe a sigh of relief, knowing that they will be spared AD for a while. A much smaller subgroup will know that AD is probably on their horizon. It is difficult to argue that such foreknowledge for those more likely to manifest AD is anything but an added burden of anxiety, even if support groups are available. Moreover, even in this subgroup the predictive value is limited. Why not let current diagnostic testing for AD in its very early clinical phase suffice? By a process of exclusion of other causes, it is considered 80 to 90 percent accurate, and the mild phase of AD will last several years (unless progression is unusually rapid), allowing people with the diagnosis to fulfill some dreams and make executive plans. In one case, for example, the family of a woman diagnosed with probable AD drove across New England in autumn to see the colors, something they had planned to do later on.

It may be more beneficial for Americans to resist the desire for presymptomatic foreknowledge and enjoy their later years, knowing that the power of the mind will diminish, for some more than others. When clinical signs of AD are present, most people know that something is wrong, are diagnosed, and struggle to adjust. There is no benefit in making this struggle more protracted. Only if preventive measures are clearly validated and available does having foreknowledge make much sense. To date, there are no such measures, though this may change if research progresses. Until then, elderly people should enjoy life one day at a time and not be preoccupied with diseases for which they show no symptoms, the victims of a hypergenetic culture.

Yet the principle work in presymptomatic testing is not in neuropsychology but in the area of genetic susceptibility testing. This chapter introduces in nontechnical style the emerging research on the genetics of AD in relation to ethical questions surrounding presymptomatic susceptibility testing and prenatal testing, although currently the main application of AD genetics is in confirming diagnosis. The field of AD genetics is in a period of intense research; information must still be gathered before most people can be counseled with clarity. As distinct forms of familial AD inheritance are differentiated, genetic testing will become a significant area of ethical discussion.

But I qualify this discussion with previously stated concerns about the dominance of biomedical data in our culture, which has imposed a medical model of reality on the journey into old age. The well-being and happiness of an old person should not be held hostage to data that offer no clear benefit and may create limitations and burdens. How much should fear of dementia shape the medicalized lives of the elderly, allowing rule by "genocrats" whose main function in this case is to label the self with complex probabilities and susceptibilities that then further contribute to the explosion of dubious medical management by "pharmocrats"? If prenatal diagnosis is intended to control the gates of life, amniocentesis for the elderly is intended to control the gates of death as the elderly seek and await information and "preinformation" in a culture of tentative aging and illusory separation from the repugnant ranks of the forgetful.

Sensationalism and Accuracy

It is important that the value of AD genetic testing, which for the most part lacks both *sensitivity* (the probability that the test will be positive in someone who will eventually manifest AD), and *specificity* (the probability that the test will be negative in someone who will not manifest AD), not be exaggerated. Public expectations are raised by the media attention given to any scientific work on genetics—attention consisting of the confusing sound bite that usually gives the wrong impression. There is also a culturally pervasive acceptance of "genetic determinism" that attaches more significance to the genetic factors in disease than is appropriate. Therefore researchers in AD genetics must be careful about how they convey information to the public. While researchers can and should announce their findings, they must not overstate the practical significance of their data.

It is likely, however, that even the most cautious researchers will find their data fueling a certain public hysteria for a presymptomatic genetic susceptibility test that can tell individuals whether they are likely to manifest AD long before they do. By all anecdotal reports, the telephones of AD centers and clinics around the United States and Canada often ring with inquiries about "the" genetic test that can guarantee a happy retirement. People long for the miracle predictive test that might promise them full safety as they grow old. This rage for knowledge and data is like prenatal amniocentesis in which prospective parents wish to be certain that their child will be perfectly healthy. Of course experts in amniocentesis had to educate consumers to understand that this technology can eliminate specific genetic risks but cannot guarantee health.

The Amniocentesis of Old Age

Some elderly people are so formed by a hypercognitive society that first and foremost they need security from dementing illness. AD predictive testing is the amniocentesis of old age. Although its results remain for the most part vague, it nevertheless serves the psychological desire (as distinct from need) for greater certitude. Each time another rumor of a preventive measure is circulated, the value of susceptibility testing goes up dramatically.

Unlike Huntington disease (HD), another dementing illness, in which international testing guidelines are accepted and a small, designated set of families are at risk, in AD there are no accepted guidelines as of yet, and the number of people likely to request testing is extremely large. Some of the questions pertaining to genetics and late-onset dementing illnesses have already been looked at in HD. AD, however, is very different from HD, which has a mean age of onset of 38 years, is limited to a very narrow population, and has obvious physiological impact from the outset. AD is of later onset than HD and appears ubiquitous in its sporadic form; its victims are generally physiologically normal and even vigorous for years as the dementia develops.

Studies have shown for some time that first-degree relatives of persons with AD are at increased risk for developing the disease, suggesting a "familial" form (FAD) and a "sporadic" form (Heston et al., 1981). The possibility of a familial form of AD was suggested as early as 1925 and later in 1934 (Lowenberg and Waggoner, 1934). Researchers have now identified regions of at least three different chromosomes that are associated with familial cases of AD (Roses et al., 1992). Much more sporadic AD is now thought to be familial.

AD rose from obscurity in the late 1960s as studies in England showed that most dementia in elderly people is due not to cerebral atherosclerosis but rather to the same degenerative brain lesions that Alois Alzheimer described as "presenile" (arising before the arbitrary age of 65) dementia in 1907 (Blessed, Tomlinson, and Roth, 1968). A significant social movement based on alliances between family caregivers, health professionals, and research scientists moved AD from the ranks of "an obscure, rarely applied medical diagnosis to characterization as the fourth or fifth leading cause of death in the United States" (Fox, 1989). Costs in the United States for diagnosis, management, and caring for AD patients are now estimated at "well over $80 billion annually" (Selkoe, 1992). Against this background, AD genetics has become a major public concern, further intensified by the constant flow of media reports on genetic findings related to many other diseases.

The ethics arise, however, in the implementation of genetic testing: how can harms be minimized and benefits maximized? Ethical questions have not yet been systematically articulated because AD genetics is a recent development (limited in most aspects to the last eight years), and testing is just being explored. Some argue that predictive testing should only be made available if preventive intervention is possible, but benefits are said to extend beyond this because some people want information with which to make good life decisions. They want to plan for retirement and do some of the traveling now that they would have done later, in addition to wanting certainty (which cannot be delivered) for its own sake.

Burdens of testing include the potential for discrimination in employment or insurance coverage and adverse reactions such as preemptive suicide or depression. The possibility for such reactions in the context of HD gave rise to internationally accepted ethics guidelines that deal with informed consent, psychological assessment, pre- and posttest genetic counseling, identification of an individual to be present with the tested individual when results are disclosed, and screening for major psychiatric illnesses that would preclude testing, among others. With regard to HD, most people who find out their genetic risk cope reasonably well with proper support, although there has been one suicide in the United States and another in Canada.

The public needs to know how to understand and interpret AD susceptibility testing. Emerging information that makes late-onset and sporadic AD appear more familial and gene-related creates considerable public interest. How could susceptibility testing contribute to diagnostic improvement, and could any available interventions slow the onset of disease? As with HD, there may be many people who have no interest in presymptomatic testing.

If current susceptibility screening is ever developed to accuracy and testing for AD becomes more widespread, the Alzheimer's Association and other support groups should function as major conduits of information for affected families and individuals. However, tests for AD susceptibility are as of yet inadequate to justify presymptomatic testing, although testing may be used to help confirm an ambiguous diagnosis.

Current Genetic Knowledge

To avoid a technical genetic jargon that would likely offend many readers, I wish to briefly summarize what is known about AD and genetics.

Of primary public interest, the apolipoprotein (ApoE) gene is found on chromosome 19. The initial clinical ApoE genetic testing programs to further confirm the AD risk associated with combinations of the ApoE alleles is in full swing in both the United States and Canada. This gene contains the instructions enabling the body to make a protein called apolipoprotein E. The best known function of apolipoprotein is to transport cholesterol into cells, although other functions are just beginning to be discovered. Researchers have long known that the ApoE gene has three slightly different forms (technically, "alleles"), of which each individual has a combination of two (E2, E3, and E4), producing slightly different proteins. The proteins produced by the different gene forms show apparent differences in function.

The identification of the ApoE4 form as a major risk factor for AD may be used as an aid to clinical diagnosis. It may also become a presymptomatic test for AD. In 1991 the Duke group led by Allen D. Roses, M.D., made the claim that "late-onset" (mean age of onset greater than 65 years) AD was associated with chromosome 19. In late 1992 and early 1993, the Duke group announced that the ApoE4 gene form is more than three times as common in patients with late-onset AD, regardless of family history. Hence, the E4 gene variant was proposed as the first concrete biological risk factor for late-onset AD.

A genetic risk factor (susceptibility gene) is different from a (causative) disease gene because it only indicates the *likelihood* of developing the disease. Many people with AD do not have the ApoE4 gene. While people with the ApoE4 gene appear to be at increased risk for AD, it is difficult to be specific about the extent of that increase in all populations, although knowledge is growing rapidly and in some populations it is possible to be fairly precise. Strittmatter et al. found a frequency for the E4 gene of 16 percent among controls (people with no familial history of AD), compared with 50 percent in those from families in which late-onset AD has been identified (Strittmatter et al., 1993). In studies of Corder et al., it was concluded that the overall risk of AD by age 75 is near certainty for individuals with the E4-E4 genotype, and threefold greater for individuals with one E4 allele than for those with none (Corder et al., 1993; Saunders et al., 1993). Another study indicates that one reason for higher AD susceptibility, in addition to the presence of the E4 form, is the absence of the E2 gene, which has a protective effect. In other words, the two gene forms have opposite effects: E4 contributes to AD susceptibility while E2 protects (Corder et al., 1994). Researchers across the United States and in other countries are actively pursuing epidemiological studies to clarify genetic risk associated with different combinations of ApoE genes. Predictive value is still to be reconfirmed.

The ApoE development is especially interesting because it makes genetic susceptibility testing relevant to a large population of people, in contrast to a clear set of families as is the case with HD. The demand for screening may be tremendous. One study concludes that the 90-year lifetime risk for AD among first-degree relatives is about 50 percent, again suggesting that much more AD is genetic and familial than has been previously assumed. This study indicates that it is now common for relatives of AD patients to inquire about their own risk (Breitner, 1991). Predictive screening based on the ApoE gene may identify those who would benefit from drugs that would prevent or weaken the bond with amyloid, if such drugs can be developed, or possibly from currently available drugs such as tacrine (Cognex).

There is another development in AD genetics that will affect almost no one, and therefore will be only mentioned here in passing. In 1987 it was reported that some families with high rates of AD have a genetic error on chromosome 21 (St. George-Hyslop et al., 1987; St. George-Hyslop et al., 1990). For technical reasons, genetic testing is difficult (Karlinsky et al., 1991). Yet the most recent developments in familial AD (FAD) genetics do make predictive testing an immediate possibility for some families. The chromosome 21 gene mutation was confirmed in eight or more families around the world, including one in Japan, indicating that while FAD is genetically heterogeneous, this mutation is a significant cause in some families (Naruse et al., 1991). In all these families, the age of onset is roughly between 50 and 60 years. They are loosely termed early-onset FAD (mean age of onset 60 years or less). People who are past age 60 need have no worries about FAD, and anyone with such a family would surely be aware of the problem on the basis of family history.

Virtually no one, outside of a very few families throughout the world, is concerned with the chromosome 21 data (Boller et al., 1992). Yet the chromosome 21 gene was the first identified mutation and provides the initial example of the applicability of AD genetic testing, although it is almost certainly not the most important mutation. Early-onset FAD (in rare cases diagnosed in patients as young as their midthirties) associated with the gene mutation on chromosome 21 may affect some small percentage of all AD patients (at most 1 percent). Whatever the percentage, the National Alzheimer's Association indicates that families of AD patients are concerned with new genetic findings and that genetic questions to health care professionals "will likely be asked more frequently" (Williams, 1993). This overconcern with genetics is a growing cultural problem.

Finally, in 1992 research teams reported a region of chromosome 14 linked to an unusually early onset FAD, with age of onset before 50 years (Mullan et al., 1992; Schellenberg et al., 1992). While the chromosome 14 gene has yet to be identified, it seems to be linked in many more families than chromosome 21–related FAD, and therefore may be more important with regard to potential genetic testing.

Ethical Issues

There are a number of ethical issues that pertain to genetic presymp-tomatic testing and often to psychological tests such as Masur's. In this section, an overview of these issues is provided. There is no pretension of full resolution, which awaits social debate.

Justice and Allocation

The likely magnitude of AD susceptibility testing programs raises issues of justice and allocation. Will everyone whose relatives have had AD think himself or herself susceptible? If much more AD is familial than was previously assumed, the distinction between sporadic AD and FAD blurs, creating a demand for testing much greater than that for Hunting-ton disease. With HD, a clearly defined group of families exists, and therefore the wider public is not involved; however, with AD, information on genetics is likely to affect a much wider population, especially when the distinctions between familial and sporadic forms are difficult to com-municate and less than clear-cut. Providing genetic counseling services for HD does not greatly strain resources, but we can expect resources to be strained by genetic testing for widespread diseases such as AD (Nolan and Swenson, 1988).

AD genetics raises questions of resources, access, and justice. Would genetic screening for AD be included in a basic health care package avail-able to all citizens, although no preventive lifestyle modifications are yet pos-sible (unless the questionable claim that mental activity is AD-preventive can be verified)? If the full genetic testing and proper counseling costs per person are estimated conservatively at a thousand dollars, the total costs could quickly rise.

The question of justice is complicated by the fact that partially preven-tive pharmacological agents may be found. The experience with tacrine sug-gests that patients in the earliest stages of AD are likely to benefit most be-fore extensive neuronal death has accumulated. If effective AD therapies became available and early treatment prevented neuronal cell death, this would be reason to screen early and widely and to consider screening a valu-able use of resources. It is likely that with therapies available, the relative pri-ority of AD testing in a just health care system would rise greatly. Should the individual pay for testing or should it be covered by insurance? As AD genetic testing unfolds, do people have a right to the knowledge yielded? What cost qualifications might limit this right?

Presymptomatic Screening and Disclosure

Presymptomatic screening raises serious ethical issues regarding pre- and posttest counseling and support. In a recent article entitled "Should Patients with Alzheimer's Disease Be Told Their Diagnosis?" the authors regard it as ethically valid to withhold from patients, even those able to comprehend, information about diagnosis and prognosis (Drickamer and Lachs, 1992). Some physicians and other health care workers, as well as many family members, fear that telling the truth will cause distress to patients, that they will feel stigmatized, become depressed even to the point of despair, and become more difficult to manage. These concerns are not entirely unwarranted.

However, disclosing presymptomatic genetic test results to the affected person with the assurance that counseling and other services will be available, including participation in support groups, frequently allows for an emotional adjustment. There is an ethical obligation to ensure that the anxiety and fears of those with positive test results are properly attended to. Disclosing positive test results allows the person to participate as far as possible in the development of a plan of action for the future, but should genetic tests be available to people even in young adulthood? Clearly a genetic test that brings bad news can lead to harm in the absence of a support system. The content, timing, and manner of disclosure must be appropriate and sensitive. A significant danger of presymptomatic testing in the absence of ethical guidelines is that information will be irresponsibly disclosed and result in adverse reactions.

Presymptomatic testing is complicated in the case of AD because this disease is on the cutting edge of the national and international debate over physician-assisted suicide, as I will discuss in chapter 8. While it is true that requests for suicide from the terminally ill are often shaped by untreated pain and inadequate psychosocial conditions, what of requests by people with a presymptomatic diagnosis of a progressive dementia that will ultimately lead to the loss of memory?

It is critical to emphasize that the next decade or two will bring dramatic advances in our understanding of the etiology of AD and thus in disease prevention. Presumably many researchers would not countenance preemptive suicide and would emphasize the likelihood of future therapies. Nevertheless, there is a temporal gap between the availability of testing and of therapies.

People fear the loss of memory in AD and may not respond positively to the experienced clinician who counsels the individual who has received news of a positive presymptomatic test to "take it one day at a time." Such concerns merit concerted proactive moral deliberations.

How can people who are at high genetic risk for AD be properly supported? What forms of counseling should be available to the tested individual before and after testing? What is the most sensitive way to disclose testing results to avoid adverse reaction? What access to data should family members have, if any? This must be frankly addressed in relation to presymptomatic testing.

In view of the dementing characteristics shared by AD and Huntington disease, both of which are incurable neurodegenerative diseases, it is prudent to consider predictive testing programs for AD in the light of the HD experience. Therefore, a first step is to review current HD testing protocols and the genetics of AD to consider the extent to which existing predictive testing programs designed for HD can be utilized and modified for AD testing programs. This is a logical step, since much careful attention has already been devoted to ethics and HD genetic testing.

Prenatal Testing

As a general rule, people wish to have prenatal genetic testing available and feel they have a right to it, but they may not utilize it (Jedlicka-Kohler, Gotz, and Eichler, 1994). Obviously AD is a disabling disease. How will genetic counselors respond to AD testing in this context, if it occurs? One area of debate is whether prenatal testing for AD susceptibility ought to be available without the intent of selective abortion. A study of attitudes of 306 pregnant Caucasian women toward carrier screening for cystic fibrosis indicates that 98 percent of respondents think screening should be offered, that 69 percent of respondents would accept such screening themselves, and that 29 percent of respondents would terminate the pregnancy if the fetus were found to have the disease (Botkin and Alemagno, 1992). Prenatal testing for Huntington disease is not provided unless abortion would follow a positive test, largely on the grounds that this would be tantamount to imposing a presymptomatic test for the born child when such testing should be a matter of personal choice for the individual upon legal age (Corson et al., 1990). Guidelines drawn up by the International Huntington Association and the World Federation of Neurology indicate that any couple requesting prenatal testing should be aware that there is little point in taking the test if the intent is to complete the pregnancy regardless (World Federation of Neurology, 1989). A revision of these guidelines asserts this even more strongly. What limitations, if any, should be placed on prenatal testing in order not to violate "the child's right not to know if in fact the pregnancy is brought to term" (Karjala, 1992)?

We need to develop ethics guidelines for ApoE susceptibility testing (e.g., informed consent, pre- and posttest genetic counseling, potential controversy over prenatal counseling, when should testing be available and to whom).

The possibilities of prenatal FAD testing and selective abortion raise important humanistic and ethical questions that genetic counselors, women, families, and society must grapple with. While selective abortion is an old topic, the genome project raises it anew (Post et al., 1992). Granted the legal right to elective abortion, of which the right to selective abortion is a subset, it is still timely to consider the moral underpinnings of the choices that women and couples can freely make. In this area of ethical concern, decisions will also be influenced by possible new treatments on the horizon.

Prenatal testing for HD is available, and presumably it will be for FAD. Will such technologies create "a rise in the standards of production for children," establishing "a set of norms of acceptability, and then narrow, and narrow, and narrow yet again those norms" (Rothman, 1986)? Some argue that the medical profession should abandon a position of ethical neutrality with regard to prenatal sex selection, partly because it sets precedents for selection unrelated to disease or disability (Wertz and Fletcher, 1989). Obviously AD is a disabling disease. But does prenatal testing for such a late-onset disease raise unique moral questions?

In the absence of any obviously grave and immediately threatening defect, vexing decisions will be made based on the severity, probability, and age at onset of disease or disability. AD can be compared with Turner syndrome, for instance, which affects girls, resulting in shortness, infertility, and often odd appearance. Yet life expectancy is normal, and with in vitro fertilization it has become possible for some of those with Turner syndrome to have babies. The probability of occurrence is clear, as is the age of onset, but the severity of the syndrome might not be considered great. The difficulty, ethically, comes with parental decisions about the acceptability of the child's quality of life. What shall we do with the freedom to decide, especially when genetic conditions have variable expressivity from mild to serious, have variable likelihood of manifestation, are variable as to the age at onset, and may be treatable? Is a disease such as AD sufficient moral (in contrast to legal) grounds for selective abortion, even though the eventual sufferer will have many decades of good and unimpaired living?

There are several humanistic themes to be considered in relation to the question regarding the suffering of offspring. First, parents rightfully prefer not to bring lives filled with suffering into the world. Few, if any, would quarrel with the assumption that it is preferable to have healthy children who are not born into physical pain. When prenatal diagnosis reveals a grave defect that makes life an onerous burden of suffering, the principle "do no harm" may for many but certainly not all parents morally justify abortion. But is it wrong to assume that suffering is the necessary result of every genetic defect or that lives with degrees of physical suffering cannot be creative and meaningful? How does our concept of suffering relate to concepts of the quality of life (to be discussed in chapter 7), which always contain some subjective element, except in the most severe circumstances of neurological impairment (Asch, 1989, p. 320)?

A second broad humanistic theme is human contingency. The word "contingency" refers to a chance event beyond human control, and there was no control over the genetic quality of the newborn. Our desire not to bring imperfection into the world must be tempered by a recognition that suffering brought about by events we can never control is an ineradicable part of life. Those who are genotypically and phenotypically more "perfect" than others can lead tragic lives, brought about by unforeseen circumstances. Contingency is at the very heart of human experience, and it has been a classical function of religious worldviews to make sense of this. Does genetic technology foster a will to control that prevents our coming to grips with the basic reality of contingency from which we never escape?

A third humanistic theme focuses on images of human perfection. All perfectionism must be tempered by an awareness of what Leslie A. Fiedler called "the tyranny of the normal" (1985, p. 151). Fiedler notes a "deep ambivalence toward fellow creatures who are perceived at any given moment as disturbingly deviant, outside currently acceptable physiological norms." One of the ways in which persons who depart from "normals" (e.g., people with dementia in a hypercognitive culture) contribute to the community is by challenging us to overcome social stigmas and to accept difference in our midst, including the lives of the deeply forgetful. People who are different and "imperfect" teach us about the meaning of equality and commitment. But we are beings who fear difference, so diversity is hard to sustain. The very nature of human perfection has, of course, been the subject of acrimonious debate over the centuries. How circumspect should we be about declaring too imperfect those who must endure somewhat earlier in life the very neurological frailty some believe eventually may assault a great many of us if we live long enough? There is limited societal interest in questioning selective abortion for grave genetic defects that will manifest immediately or early in life (Faden et al., 1987). Selective abortion for diseases that will manifest later in life, however, raises greater concern. Hypothetically, what of a fetus with a 64 percent probability of AD with onset at age 68?

Any decision regarding prenatal AD testing is complicated by the possibility that therapies may eventually be available to slow the progression of the disease and that environments may be developed that enhance the quality of life for the AD patient. The woman or couple considering selective abortion for a child who might manifest AD later in life must ponder possibilities for future medical and environmental amelioration of dementia.

Long-Term Care Insurance

It will be important to address the potential impact of susceptibility testing on private long-term care insurance industry (est. 2 million policies currently in effect affordable to an est. 20 percent of population). Those who know they are at higher risk for AD will want to buy insurance. With regulations possible that will restrict insurance companies from requesting genetic information, this industry may disappear due to adverse selection. Policy questions in this context, especially regarding confidentiality of susceptibility test results, will be addressed.

In the last five years, private long-term care insurance has become a fast-growing product in the insurance market. Unless prohibited by law, it seems likely that private insurers would want to have new applicants for private long-term care insurance undergo AD genetic testing. It has been argued that genetic-risk data ought not to be allowed as a qualification for insurance coverage. While this argument might have merit for general health care coverage, does it apply to targeted coverage, such as long-term care insurance? Is it fair to prohibit insurers from using AD genetic data when the problem of adverse selection might otherwise be devastating? As Robert Cook-Deegan wrote two years ago, "Just imagine the problems if it became possible to detect genetic predisposition to Alzheimer's disease in a substantial fraction of cases, for example. This alone would completely wipe out the possibility of a private market for long-term care insurance" (Cook-Deegan, 1994).

Envoi

As our understanding of the genetics, etiology, and possible therapy of AD develops in the decades ahead, the ethical quandaries surrounding presymptomatic and other testing will come increasingly to the fore. Given the phenomenon of the "aging society" in industrialized societies around the world, these quandaries will meet with various responses in the light of varying worldviews and presuppositions, and they will challenge us ethically to distinguish between the universal and the relative. As the U.S. health care system becomes increasingly global in its patient population, some cross-cultural variation can be anticipated. The extent to which we will build moral consensus on these issues remains to be seen. However, there is no question that AD genetics will be at the cutting edge of the "genethics" discussion as knowledge progresses and increasing numbers of patients make inquiries in the clinical setting. Current progress in AD genetics research is of course laudatory but may or may not give rise to therapeutic innovations. But meanwhile, we must guard vigilantly against the irresponsible introduction of genetic testing and work to establish clinical guidelines consistent with the principles of "do no harm."

The public should not be swept up by "genocracy," as though the beginnings of genetic analysis of AD has much to offer of immediate benefit. The genetics can provide some degree of foreknowledge regarding susceptibility for some subgroups, but it offers neither certainty nor current medical cure. Genetics is like a genie that can be used for good or ill and that has limited powers to impact or remove the experience of dementia from our aging society, although its powers may grow with the passage of time. AD genetics is not yet a medical miracle, but it already creates many moral muddles. Importantly, Dr. Allen D. Roses indicates clearly that ApoE genetic testing is useful *only* in confirming a diagnosis, not in providing predictive information.

SEVEN

✤ Quality of Life, Treatment Burdens, and the Right to Comfort

Few topics are more contentious in biomedical ethics than "quality of life," fueling as it has at least three decades of philosophical, theological, anthropological, and clinical debate. For those in some cultural and religious traditions, treatment limitations based on "poor" quality of life violate the principle of the sanctity of life, according to which all human life is sacred, inviolable, and worthy of preserving with whatever medical technology might be available; "quality" considerations are therefore viewed as morally dangerous, subjecting people with progressive dementia to the cultural tyranny of rationality and productivity. As Sidney Callahan states, "After all, who gets to decide, for whom, and by what standards? Cannot quality of life be interpreted in a prejudicial fashion and abused by powerful elites? If we give up the idea of the sanctity and inviolability of bodily life, then a traditional taboo is broken, a wedge is opened for powerful interests to extinguish the demented, ill, immature, aged, or other vulnerable undesirables who cannot defend themselves" (1992, p. 138).

While Callahan believes that quality of life should be afforded moral significance when it reaches an extremely low level such as with the anencephalic infant, she is very cautious about considerations of quality because it contains an irreducibly subjective element, even though she does think that we must cross this Rubicon.

In response to the tyranny of elites, some reassert the principle of sanctity as a veneer of protection: all human life is equally valuable regardless of quality. The practical outcome of this position is a medical vitalism, that is, so long as the body lives on, no matter how stripped the self is of relational capacity, human life must be preserved. After all, it is commonly asserted, how can we "normals" fairly judge the highly subjective quality of another human being's life? One philosopher has gone so far as to liken people with severe dementia to dogs, since they supposedly "lack capacities for hopes and fears, dreads and longings for their futures" (Brock, 1993, p. 372). This is an offensive simplification, since people with severe dementia generally do have fears and longings, even if these are limited to the immediate present.

We must be more cautious than Brock regarding quality-of-life judgments and dementia. Let me play the role of pure provocateur by asserting what must surely be a partly offensive statement: many people with progressive dementia, once reaching the point of forgetting forgetfulness, are spared most human anxieties. No longer must the person grapple with the fear of death, for death is itself forgotten. Such deeply forgetful minds are disengaged and liberated from the cares and burdens that drive so many of us to despair and sometimes to corruption. The person's attention is fixed on a colorful flower that is forever new and therefore fascinating. It is possible to wander on the same path day after day, and it never gets old. There is a detachment from the things of the world, from possessiveness, that mimics the wisdom of some of Dostoyevsky's slightly demented exemplars of virtue, such as the old serf Makar Evanovich Dolgoruky, about whom one observer notes: "Moreover, I'm sure I'm not just imagining things if I say that at certain moments he looked at me with a strange, even uncanny love" (Dostoyevsky, 1988, p. 221). Historians point out that medieval and Renaissance Christianity, in theory if less so in practice, saw madness as sometimes holy: "A faith founded upon the madness of the Cross, which crusaded against worldliness, which lauded the innocence of the infant, which valued the spiritual mysteries of contemplation, asceticism and the mortification of the flesh, and prized faith over intellect, could not help but see gleams of godliness in the simplicity of the fool" (Porter, 1989, p. 14).

Jonathan Swift, in his *Gulliver's Travels* (1727), described the "struldbrugs" among the Luggnaggian people:

> They have no remembrance of anything but what they learned and observed in their youth and middle age, and even that is imperfect. And for the truth or particulars of any fact, it is safer to depend on common traditions than upon their best recollections. The least miserable among them appear to be those who turn to dotage, and entirely lose their memories; these meet with more pity and assistance, because they want many bad qualities which abound in others (1945, pp. 214–215).

Other struldbrugs are miserable, "dead to all natural affection." They all, after reaching 90, "forget the common appellation of things, and the names of persons, even those who are their nearest friends and relations" (Swift, 1945, p. 215). Nor can they amuse themselves with reading, "because their memory will not serve to carry them from the beginning of a sentence to the end" (p. 215). Eventually, they are unable to hold any conversation, "and thus lie under the disadvantage of living like foreigners in their own country" (p. 215). Struldbrugs receive a scanty public allowance; they are "despised and hated by all sorts of people" (p. 216).

Four years later, in 1731, Swift wrote his most famous poem, entitled "Verses on the Death of Dr. Swift, D.S.P.D.," in which he may have anticipated his own eventual dementia, but was more likely drawing on his observations of others:

> Yet, thus methinks, I hear 'em speak;
> See, how the Dean begins to break;
> Poor gentleman, he droops apace,
> You plainly find it in his face:
> That old vertigo in his head,
> Will never leave him, till he's dead:
> Besides, his memory decays,
> He recollects not what he says;
> He cannot call his friends to mind;
> Forgets the place where last he dined:
> Plies you with stories o'er and o'er,
> He told them fifty times before. (1993, p. 152)

The poem concludes, "He gave the little wealth he had, / To build a house for fools and mad" (1993, p. 165).

Swift, dean of St. Patrick's Cathedral, Dublin, willed that his estate be used to fund the building of a home for the "fools and mad." This place of care, known as St. Patrick's Hospital, opened in Dublin in 1745, the year of his death, and is still open to this day. Swift had insisted on three conditions: that the institution be situated to enable family members to visit; that there be no display of residents for the amusement of the public; and that it be located near a general hospital.

Given Swift's problems with vertigo, it is possible that he suffered from Ménière's disease. He was demented and described his memory loss years before his death, although the cause of his dementia remains unknown. The last five years of his life were marked by eccentricities, combative behavior, depression, and severe dementia. A satirist as well as an Anglican clergyman, he long manifested "infinite distress for the insane" who (Dennis, 1964, p. 138), like struldbrugs, were "despised and hated by all sorts of people." He bequeathed his wealth to enhance the quality of life of the deeply forgetful.

Swift's legacy instructs us today that even if we appeal to quality of life in moral deliberations about the fate of people with dementia, we must be very cautious because our assessment of quality may be unduly low, thereby diminishing our moral resolve to enhance the lives of the most vulnerable among us. Yet with due caution, I do think that quality of life has moral significance in cases of advanced dementia and that we must guard against vitalism.

In this chapter, I will argue that the most significant quality-of-life concern must be with the burdens that life-extending treatment can impose on many people with dementia. It is thus often humane to decide against treatments that are intended for other than palliative purposes, although palliative comfort care may have the side effect of extending life. In arguing against the inhumane extension of life, I by no means compromise my ethic of radically equal moral standing for people with dementia.

It is my view that the quality of life and the sanctity of life form a beneficial dialectic. Between them, individuals, families, and society negotiate the questions of life prolongation and treatment withdrawal. Without appreciation for the sanctity of life, life can be casually and quickly cast aside in the name of cognition and privilege; without appreciation for the quality of life, especially with regard to interventions that are perceived by the person as torturous or that result in various forms of serious discomfort, life can be held hostage to medical technologies that no longer serve humanity but dominate it.

We must keep in memory an expression from the Nazi era, *lebenunwertes Leben,* "life unworthy of life," applied principally to people with mental illness or dementia; we must also remember that while both Judaism and Christianity profess that each person is created in the image of God and therefore has inherent and equal value, only minority voices in these traditions require treatment in all circumstances.

Conceptual Background: Quality and Humaneness

As medical technology advances to the point when human life can be maintained almost indefinitely, questions pertaining to the negative impact of those technologies on quality of life inevitably arise. I reject the move of ethicists who have approached the definition of "quality" by specifying certain indicators of personhood that make a life valuable. Among the indicators suggested two decades ago by Joseph F. Fletcher were self-awareness, self-control, a sense of time, a sense of futurity, a sense of the past, capability to relate to others, and communication (1975). Since then, many others have asserted indicators of quality, almost all of which reflect the rationalism of their proponents. Of course these indicators apply no better to many people with dementia than they do to newborns; they provide no protection to the weak nor any assurance that people with dementia will be protected.

It is my view that the most important aspect of quality of life for people with dementia is the emotional adjustment facilitated by affirming care, as I indicated in earlier chapters. I would extend this concern with emotional adjustment to preclude treatments that create suffering. People with dementia are sentient and should be treated humanely. Acceptable quality of life for people with dementia, as I interpret it, is a matter of *(a)* adjustment to and coping with the experience of increasing forgetfulness prior to the point of forgetting that one forgets; *(b)* emotional-behavioral condition in the more advanced stages; and *(c)* avoidance of treatment-induced agitation, fear, and pain.

On the one end of the continuum, there are those with dementia who have a relatively calm emotional life punctuated by occasional facial expressions of joy (a smile in response to a touch on the shoulder); on the other end are those who do nothing but groan and scream out as though in terror or pain unless burdened by heavy sedation. Toward this second end, where the person seems continuously tormented, continued life is obviously a burden and should not be imposed by life-extending interventions. When the experience of dementia is more emotionally benign, life-extension is tolerable for the person and therefore morally acceptable but not requisite.

For people with dementia who have indicated their treatment preferences by advance directive such as a living will or by durable power of attorney for health care combined with such a will, we must honor their wishes in most cases. There may be exceptions, as when the person requests all treatment possible under any circumstances but treatments are burdensome and violate the principle of nonmaleficence. Many people, however, informed by the very hypercognitive values that characterize our culture, will indicate that were they to become severely demented they would want to let nature take its course so that death might come sooner than later. Such decisions must be honored according to autonomy and self-determination. But when the wishes of the person with dementia are not known, rough lines can be sketched with regard to the best interests of the person in accordance with emotional-behavioral condition.

The essential norm must be how the potential treatment will be likely to detract from the quality of life of the person with dementia. Would it impose considerable fear for a confused and disoriented person? There can be inhumane suffering as a result of *(a)* treatment that is interpreted by the person with dementia as assault and even torture; *(b)* the prolongation of the person's life if behavioral problems are uncontrollable or controllable only by continuous heavy sedation; *(c)* physical freedom being restricted, resulting in bedsores, infections, and other painful burdens, or *(d)* withdrawal of assent to treatment as indicated by continued attempts to pull out dialysis or feeding tubes, and the like.

Regarding inhumane treatment under type *(a)* above, David H. Smith wrote, "At a minimum I would say that dementia may have the effect that some life-sustaining treatment can only be *perceived* as torture, and that perception is a formidable argument against using them" (1992, p. 48). Erich H. Loewry wrote of the moral significance of the "suffering produced by the treatment," the recipient "may be baffled by their perception of the caring milieu turning on them" (Loewry, 1987, p. 1467). As for inhumane treatment under type *(b)* above, Nicholas Rango provided the example of the person with dementia who manifests "incorrigible acts of self-mutilation or intractable states of paranoia and hallucinations" (1985, p. 838). Regarding inhumane treatment under type *(c)* above, Rango gave the example of a person with severe multi-infarct dementia: "It is often impossible to feed, move, or lift such patients without unintentionally tormenting them" (p. 838). Under inhumane treatment *(d)* above, Loewry wrote of "the patient's capacity for sustained understanding of treatment and cooperation with the regimen," which makes the resistance to treatment and thereby the withdrawal of assent a moral consideration (1987, p. 1467).

In summary, decisions that impose considerable burdens on the person with dementia in the name of vitalism must not and cannot be tolerated, any more than we would tolerate wanton violence or torture. There ought to be limits on the rights of individuals (through advance directives) and families (in cases of the incompetent person who has no advance directive) to demand treatments that are significantly burdensome. Some legal precedent for this ethical position has been outlined (Dresser, 1994). Such restrictions are not violations of radical equality, but reasonable implementations of standard moral rule against inflicting harm and suffering. Surrogate decisions based on a person's "best interests" must be loosely circumscribed. When the treatment experience of the person with dementia is more benign, I acknowledge extensive latitude in familial authority over levels of intervention and in the authority of advance directives (Wildes, 1994).

What are the morally appropriate levels of life-extending medical treatment for patients in the advanced stages of progressive and eventually fatal dementia such as Alzheimer disease? I have circumscribed some rough limits on treatment on the basis of inhumaneness, while avoiding most qualitative judgments. To reiterate the reasons for my conservative approach on "quality," *(a)* quality of life is partly contingent on the extent to which a supportive environment is created to enhance well-being and is thus a self-fulfilling prophecy, since quality of life is dependent in crucial ways on the attitudes and actions of caregivers; *(b)* a reliable qualitative measure of a patient's internal experience is impossible, since quality of life has a subjective aspect that no outward observer can assess; and *(c)* quality of life might be misused to rid society of unproductive members. Yet my desire for a categorical prohibition of inhumane treatments is qualitative and would doubtless affect considerable numbers of people with advanced dementia. My concern is with the iatrogenic imposition of psychic and physical suffering in the context of a vulnerable population such as people with dementia who are easily captured by technology.

The Physician Perspective on Quality of Life

Those who embrace a wider notion of quality of life than do I may attach moral significance to the loss of capacities to make judgments and solve problems; to remember recent events; to remember past events; to handle business, financial and/or social affairs; to pursue hobbies and interests; to form and maintain relationships with others; to recognize close family members or friends; to recognize oneself; to plan for the future; to eat; to control bladder and bowel; and to communicate through speech. The fact that all of these capacities may eventually be lost to people with profound and terminal dementia explains why there is certainly as much fear of Alzheimer disease as of terminal cancer or other diseases.

In clinical discussions regarding treatment limitation, with people with mild dementia or with patient surrogates, reference to quality of life is not uncommon. Since physician perspectives inevitably influence medical decision making, it is important to understand any physician consensus on this issue.

My interest in physician attitudes regarding quality of life and its moral significance, if any, in no way questions the right of people with dementia or their surrogates to participate in making decisions and to have determining authority. Implementation of this right among the elderly continues to be a topic of considerable empirical investigation (Diamond et al., 1989; Zweibel and Cassel, 1989). Yet such a right does not preclude the physician from expressing his or her moral conscience, nor should it. It is an error to think that patient autonomy requires the physician to abandon his or her moral agency, reduced thereby to a technician whose only function is to obey patients or surrogates even in cases where treatment appears futile and therefore unconscionable to the physician (Miles, 1991).

Attention to physician views is justified, since most clinical decisions occur in the context of discussion between doctor and patient or surrogates, and decisions are therefore partly shaped by physician values. It is beneficence, not authoritarianism, that prompted Ingelfinger to argue that physicians have an obligation to respectfully recommend a course of action, rather than simply lay out the alternatives and abandon patients to isolated autonomy (1980). The physician as well as the patient has a moral voice, calling for an "ethics of communication" (Moody, 1992) in which the physician is both "a moderate autonomist and a moderate welfarist" (Pellegrino and Thomasma, 1988).

In assessing quality of life, a physician may attach great significance to loss of relational capacity or may take a less relational view of quality of life on the grounds that patients lacking communicative capacities can still demonstrate underlying affective responses and may retain greater self-awareness than relational incapacities suggest (Foley, 1992). It is possible to place moral weight on the perception that no matter how incapacitated, a patient nevertheless seems relatively serene.

It is due to wide disparity of perspective regarding quality of life that within the medical community "consensus breaks down when the attempt is made to determine the nature of the therapeutic obligation to the demented patient, particularly with respect to life-sustaining treatment" (Rango, 1985). Volicer detected lack of consensus among health care professionals regarding patients in the persistent vegetative state and in people with advanced dementia (Volicer, 1986).

In a 1991 cross-national empirical study of physicians' attitudes toward life-extending treatment interventions in cases of elderly people with severe dementia, considerable disagreement was evident (Alemayehu, Molloy, and Guyatt, 1991). The authors prepared a questionnaire asking "What decisions would physicians make when confronted with a critically ill, demented elderly man?" They presented the case of an 82-year-old man with life-threatening gastrointestinal bleeding who three years earlier had been diagnosed by a neurologist as suffering from probable AD. He cannot answer a simple question coherently, but seems to understand some simple commands. His behavior is agitated; he wanders, does not recognize his daughter, and has urinary incontinence. In seven countries, physicians in academic medical centers at family practice, internal medicine, and geriatric rounds were questioned about their views on treatment levels. The authors concluded that there is wide variation of opinion both within and among countries. For example, only 6 percent of Australian physicians recommended treatment in a medical intensive care unit, whereas 32 percent of U.S. physicians did so. Conversely, only 21 percent of Australian physicians chose supportive care, compared with only 3 percent of U.S. physicians.

The variation that this study found is difficult to interpret. No information is provided about the reasons underlying physician perspectives, the level of physician training, or the availability of technology. There was no attempt made to vary the severity of dementia to identify those points along the continuum of decline that physicians might consider morally significant with respect to aggressiveness of treatment. Along this continuum, in the absence of any advance directive or known family members and with assurance of no legal action against the physician, would pneumonia be treated with antibiotics, CPR be provided in the event of an arrest, or artificial nutrition provided if required?

With advance directives present and clearly indicated to physicians in a study of end-stage events among elderly nursing home residents, physicians not infrequently decided that there was no benefit to be gained for the patient from aggressive treatments. The authors conclude that in caring for incapacitated elderly patients, "physicians balance respect for autonomy with other competing ethical principles in order to make what they believe are the wisest decisions" (Danis et al., 1991). In this particular study, the tendency of nursing-home physicians was to ignore advance directives calling for aggressive treatment or transfer to hospital when they thought that desired interventions such as cardiopulmonary resuscitation were contrary to the patient's welfare. This occurred in 18 of 96 end-stage events.

Clearly physician perspectives on quality of life do enter into clinical practice with the incapacitated elderly, and these perspectives therefore deserve considerable analysis. A major study of perception of quality of life indicates that with patients 65 years and older who were neither demented nor terminally ill but had at least one chronic disease, physicians consistently perceived quality of life to be lower than that indicated by the patients themselves (Pearlman and Uhlmann, 1988). This conclusion does not directly pertain to dementia patients, but it suggests a cautious attitude toward assessing the quality of life of others.

I believe that the view of quality of life that I adhere to, namely, humane treatment that categorically precludes the imposition of mental or physical pain no matter for whom and how it is requested, would be agreed to by most thoughtful physicians devoted to the arts of healing and palliation. Those physicians who hold to cognitivist theories of quality of life go a step further. They are free to inform people with dementia and their families about their ethics and to treat those who are in agreement with their position. Prospective recipients of physician care who view emotional adjustment as the central factor in quality of life may pursue another physician. The more open discussion there is about quality of life, the better.

Consensus Building: The One and the Many

The concept of quality of life is extremely complex because of the objective (external observations)-subjective (internal self-perceptions) axis (Birren and Dieckman, 1991; Walter and Shannon, 1990). Several philosophers have recently argued that as dementia progresses in severity, only supportive care is morally fitting.

Dan Brock asks, "What health care and expenditure of resources on health care is owed on grounds of justice to the severely demented elderly" (Brock, 1988)? He concentrates on the effects of dementia such as the erosion of memory and other cognitive functions that "ultimately destroy personal identity." This loss implies, for Brock, that the "severely demented have lost an interest in treatment whose ultimate purpose is to prolong or sustain lives." They retain, however, an interest in comfort, so that a painful tumor might be removed for palliative reasons.

Daniel Callahan points out that for the patient who is severely demented, "On the one hand, he has lost his capacity for reason and usually—but not always—human interaction. On the other hand, there will be no clear ground for believing that the capacity to experience emotions has been lost" (Callahan, 1987). Callahan's conclusion is that "death need not be resisted."

I am closer to Callahan's view that there are no grounds to assume the loss of emotional life. Brock's inattention to noncognitive features of quality of life, coupled with his statements about the destruction of personal identity (suggesting more knowledge of the experience of dementia than is warranted by available evidence), are noteworthy. Both prominent philosophical ethicists, Callahan and Brock conclude that purposefully life-extending treatments are uncalled for once dementia reaches a threshold of severity.

Whether the views of Brock and Callahan suggest an emerging consensus is unclear. Yet discussions have matured regarding the moral justification for medical interventions with respect to quality and quantity of life and regarding the justice of denying access to "futile" medical interventions (Truog, Brett, and Frader, 1992). Many physicians do not wish to be required to provide interventions that appear futile (Tomlinson and Brody, 1990). A physician writes that "the family cannot demand that physicians continue to give treatment that is not in the patient's best personal medical interest" (Cranford, 1991). The goals of medicine, it is argued, are comfort, palliation, and the restoration of health. Given these goals, it may be difficult for nonvitalists to defend aggressive treatment for people with advanced dementia, although I am willing to tolerate such treatment so long as it does not become inhumane.

This attitude of toleration is based on preliminary data indicating that a considerable majority of elderly nursing home residents would want only comfort care and palliation in the event of advanced AD, but a minority (an estimated 20 percent) desire aggressive life-extending treatments. This was a study using case vignettes of forty-four alert elderly nursing home residents (Michelson et al., 1991). For those in advanced stages of dementia, would it be just to impose categorical limits on the prolongation of life, except as a side effect of palliation and comfort care? This would be too draconian; limits should only be imposed at the point of reasonable judgment of inhumane results.

Consensus building in this area should focus exclusively on progressive and irreversible cognitive decline in adults who were once mentally intact and legally competent but whose disease is in its advanced stages. Yet these queries do have some relevance to people with degrees of fixed mental retardation or other cognitive impairments that present no decline from a previous more intact mental state. I consider only the primary degenerative dementias such as Alzheimer disease that eventuate in death and can therefore be reasonably understood as extended terminal illnesses. The progressive nature of Alzheimer-type dementia toward the profound and ultimately terminal stages puts it in a category distinct from nonprogressive conditions, such as mental retardation. Yet I do think that the standard of "no inhumane treatment" is applicable to people with severe retardation for whom some treatment constitutes an incomprehensible and serious burden.

As early as 1976, Robert Katzman wrote "In focusing attention on the mortality associated with Alzheimer disease, our goal is not to find a way to prolong the life of severely demented persons" (1976). Since the severity of progressive dementia occurs on a continuum, are there morally significant thresholds such as when the patient becomes mute and lacks all interactive capacities, or no longer recognizes loved ones? These thresholds will not be reached synchronously, but together they represent an objective loss of relational potential. Loved ones will often state that the patient is "no longer there." When these points are arrived at, has meaning and substance of human life deteriorated to the extent that the use of medical technologies for nonpalliative reasons becomes morally questionable?

I hold a less cognitive and language-oriented view of quality of life; I attribute value to the inner and emotional experiences of the self despite the fact of decline and believe that more self-identity may still be present in the person with dementia than meets the eye. People with very advanced dementia do often demonstrate underlying affective responses, and they sometimes have occasional windows of clarity when some self-identity surfaces. There is, after all, no absolute certainty about when deterioration in communication and short-term memory gives way to a loss of internal sense of self-identity (Gilmore, Whitehouse, Wykle, 1989).

I also think that social consensus in defining acceptable quality of life is highly unlikely, except in those cases in which the emotional-behavioral burden of continued existence is extreme. Where behavior indicates a relatively benign experience, I consider it morally acceptable to artificially prolong life if the person with dementia has not indicated any wishes to the contrary and family members desire intentional life-extending interventions, for example, for religious reasons.

In the terminal stages of progressive dementia, when the person is mute, bedridden, incontinent of bladder and bowel, with unmeasurable intellectual functions, and with death inevitable, comfort care is all that medicine should offer, since here anything more seems clearly inhumane. Comfort care means palliation only; that is, it excludes artificial nutrition and hydration, dialysis, and all other medical interventions unless necessary for the control of pain and discomfort. Some treatments, for example antibiotics, can be intended for palliation and comfort care but will extend life as an unintended side effect. It is crucial that care and respect for patients be sustained, no matter how advanced their dementia. This means that comfort care must never be withheld or withdrawn and that medical killing be avoided. People with the most advanced dementia still command basic human respect. In a degenerative, progressive, and irreversible dementia the results are uniformly fatal (Cohen, Kennedy, and Eisdorfer, 1984).

Dementia and Medical Futility

The extremely complex and often acrimonious discussion of quality of life has been obscured, even camouflaged, by the newer debate over medical futility (Truog, Brett, and Frader, 1992). In its broadest sense, futility is a medical determination that a therapy is of no value to a patient and should not be prescribed.

Futility is an attractive concept to physicians because it promises to restore some degree of moral leverage, or some veto power over unlimited patient autonomy when demands are made for treatments contrary to the moral goals of the art of medicine. Physicians are trained to restore health or liberate from pain, and some patient requests have no connection with these goals. Appeal to futility allows them to say no to those who would have than do nonbeneficial things.

Physicians are happier about the development of futility policies than are lawyers: the former are concerned in part with the patient's good objectively considered under beneficence; the latter seem interested in protecting every patient whim. Health care administrators and some policymakers are attracted to the idea of futility because they want to control excessive costs.

Definitions of futility seem to get wider and wider. They include concerns with quality of life, cost control, probabilities of failure/success, use of nonvalidated therapies, burdens to patients, and very brief prolongation of life. All these concerns go far beyond the narrow definition of "physiologically implausible," for example, interferon has no effect on stomach cancer, taxol will not prevent AD, etc.

The much discussed case of Helga Wanglie, 86, is a useful bench mark (Miles, 1991). Mrs. Wanglie was residing in a nursing home. She was admitted to a medical center for emergency treatment of dyspnea from chronic bronchiectasis. She was intubated, and attempts to wean her failed. A week later her heart stopped and she was resuscitated, leaving her in the persistent vegetative state (PVS) in which she lay for more than a year with the support of a mechanical ventilator. Her husband, on the basis of a religiously held sanctity-of-life ethics, insisted she believed in maintaining life at all costs (Cranford, 1991). The physicians, including Steven Miles, a geriatrician, took the case to court, invoking futility and physician conscience. The judge reaffirmed Mr. Wanglie's authority. Helga died three days later.

Wanglie is the mirror image of the famous Karen Ann Quinlin case. In Quinlin, the family members wanted the ventilator removed from their daughter (who was in the PVS condition) while physicians resisted; in Wanglie, physicians requested removal while the family resisted. This is a dramatic sea change that occurred in the brief period of fifteen years between Quinlin and Wanglie.

Is this resistance to so-called futility on the part of Mr. Wanglie understandable? I believe it is. Take the story the *Cleveland Plain Dealer* ran in a Sunday magazine in late 1993 on the case of a husband whose wife has been in the PVS condition for many years. He wheels her out into the nursing home TV room on Sundays to watch the Cleveland Browns games. She is on artificial feeding and sometimes requires ventilator support. They both wear the jersey of their favorite quarterback. The husband still hopes for a miracle. The story was entitled "True Love."

This story indicates that for some people, even the PVS condition does not disqualify a loved one from equal moral standing under the principle of do no harm. It further suggests that the concept of quality of life might be replaced by the quality of lives, including family members. The story may indicate a deep psychological problem with letting go of a loved one. But the bottom line is that regrettably, not everyone shares the view that the PVS patient can have no quality of life.

The Wanglie case boils down to different values regarding quality of life. The ventilator works, that is, it kept Mrs. Wanglie breathing, warm to the touch, and excreting human waste products. The ventilator is therefore not physiologically implausible. The real question has nothing to do with futility; rather, it has to do with how much someone in the PVS condition should be valued. And what of those who are severely demented or severely retarded?

I think it important that the notion of futility be defined very narrowly because otherwise it hides the real issues, such as quality of life and costs, which need to be discussed on their own terms. Futility should be reserved for that which is physiologically contraindicated. The dictionary definition of futility is "producing no effect." It is distorting to let the concept of futility balloon up, giving misplaced empirical concreteness to value judgments about quality of life at the end of life.

There will be considerable cross-cultural disagreement over what is futile and what is not. Some of this diversity must be accommodated in the health care setting. The effort to cram areas of tremendous cultural disparity into the so-called objective idea of futility simply cannot and will not succeed. Since this cultural disparity is generally religion-based, I wish to consider this aspect of the futility debate a little further.

Religious Caregivers, Futility, and the Sanctity of Life

What of cases in which families that strongly adhere to a sanctity-of-life vitalism insist on burdensome medical treatments that appear inhumane? In such cases, society has the duty to protect the person with advanced dementia from such interventions, including resuscitation. I allow this limit with a certain ambivalence, for I agree with the cautions of Stephen L. Carter, a prominent constitutional law scholar at Yale University. Carter argues that secular liberalism has created "a political and legal culture that presses the religiously faithful to be other than themselves, to act publicly, and sometimes privately as well, as though their faith does not matter to them" (1993, p. 3). He cites evidence for a gap between the secular minority and the largely religious U.S. population. In assessing the medical context, Carter claims that patients who refuse medical treatment for religious reasons are generally viewed with suspicion, even when tolerated. There is a tendency to pressure people to act "rationally" even if this involves their giving up religious tenets. Belief systems that are "the fundaments upon which the devout build their lives" are considered as "passing beliefs" (1993, p. 14). Carter describes the trivialization of religious belief: "Pray if you like, worship if you must, but whatever you do, do not on any account take your religion seriously" (1993, p. 15). Freedom of conscience is fine, but "privatize" your religion (do not act on it publicly), and let the secular rational consensus hold trump.

Carter points out the seriousness with which the sanctity of life and the hope for a healing are held among many Christians who reject quality-of-life determinations (1993, pp. 235–258). Intense religious conviction is a powerful force that cannot be ignored. In the Wanglie case, she was maintained on a mechanical ventilator while PVS, for reasons of religious belief. Her husband, daughter, and son insisted on this treatment because, as Steven H. Miles, Mrs. Wanglie's physician, describes, "They stated their view that physicians should not play God, that the patient would not be better off dead, that removing life support showed moral decay in our civilization, and that a miracle could occur" (1991, p. 513). Dr. Miles notes with dismay that the courts sided with the Wanglie family. Their hopes for a miracle seem to have been respected, however irrational such hopes may be.

Free exercise is justifiably overridden to promote public health; for example, medical treatment is required to minimize the spread of a contagious disease or to benefit minors, even if religious belief is offended. The free exercise clause does not sanction violation of the law: human sacrifice or other harmful actions, fraud, and behaviors deemed repulsive to basic social standards are forbidden in the religious context as they are in all other contexts. Free exercise of religion has been given wide latitude because it is invalid to limit the right of a person to act on the basis of his or her deepest and inmost convictions unless absolutely necessary. A religious rejection of medical futility judgments is neither sufficiently harmful nor socially repulsive to warrant the restriction of freedom, except when the burdens of treatment for the patient are clearly inhumane (i.e., cause pain and suffering).

Laurence H. Tribe interprets the free exercise clause as entailing a "zone of required accommodation" for those whose "religious beliefs are exceptionally burdened by a challenged state action" (1978, p. 821). Accommodation does not constitute government action in support of religion, but is rather compelled by free exercise. Violation of free exercise must be clearly justifiable in secular terms, and if limited, the interruption of religious practice must be minimized. Religious people can be exceptionally burdened by futility judgments. Christianity, particularly in more conservative churches, portrays Jesus of Nazareth as a miraculous healer. About one-fifth of the gospel material is devoted to stories of healing lepers, epileptics, the deranged, and so forth (Kelsey, 1973). The Christian conservative, like Mr. Wanglie, must construe "spiritual healing" to include more than just the mobilization of patient powers, such as laughter, courage, tenacity, and hope; it also includes the operation of a real power in the universe that can override the perceived mechanisms of the physical universe.

Even if the belief in a miracle invites instant dismissal from the legal, biomedical, and bioethics communities, the fact remains that there are believers who regard the narratives of healing as literal truths. While it is tempting to override such belief systems, the long-term impact of such disrespect for religion is cause for pause.

Wide definitions of futility include reference to time (a life will be saved for only a few days or hours), to quality of life (this person has no relational potential), probabilities of failure (CPR on an 85-year-old man with less than a 5 percent chance of surviving to discharge), costs (treatment may work, but is extremely expensive), and nonvalidation (this treatment is not yet proven effective). Narrow definitions are limited to "physiological implausibility." The only definition of futility that seems unequivocal is the narrow one, namely, treatment that is contraindicated for physiological reasons. However much one scoffs at the sanctity of life ethic, especially when coupled with hope for a miracle, it must be acknowledged that support with a mechanical ventilator kept Mrs. Wanglie breathing and was, therefore, not futile according to a narrow physiological definition.

The fallacy of misplaced concreteness must be avoided in determinations of futility, especially when it threatens religious freedom. The field of bioethics and medical law must begin to reflect more systematically on the burden that a bifurcation between conscience and action imposes on believers.

Gilbert Meilaender is a theologian for whom the sanctity of life—including bodily life—is meaningful. Meilaender wishes to "recapture the connection between our person and the natural trajectory of bodily life" (Meilaender, 1993, p. 25). He accepts the idea of medical futility with regard to the comatose person who is always highly susceptible to respiratory infections due to the impairment of cough, gag, and swallowing reflexes, and whose life span is limited to weeks or months. This is "quantitative" futility because of the improbability that treatment can preserve life. But with regard to the PVS patient, who may live for years if nourished and cared for and who has biological life without conscious autonomy, any reference to futility must be of the "qualitative" variety. His opponents would contend that when "personhood" is no longer recoverable, keeping the body animated is without benefit. But Meilaender sees moral value in the history of "the animated earth that is the body" (1993, p. 29). Human beings are "embodied creatures," embodied by divine creation, and "our person cannot be divorced from the body and its natural trajectory" (p. 32).

So Meilaender accepts quantitative futility but not qualitative futility and would preserve the bodily life of the PVS patient when many would not. His is a highly articulate and authentically held position, even if there are those who find it unpalatable. Regarding people with dementia, it is implicit that Meilaender would reject the imposition of qualitative futility judgments.

Chapter Summary

In this chapter I have made the argument that the most compelling criterion for quality of life in people with dementia is emotional-behavioral adjustment to the condition. Often, invasive medical treatments will upset this adjustment, either because such treatments cannot be understood by the recipient or because the extension of life will add to mental and physical suffering. Therefore, families, physicians, and society should deeply reflect on inhumane attempts to prolong the lives of people with dementia. This reflection does not discriminate against people with dementia; rather, it carefully considers their best interests. Although I will get overly detailed here, I accept the general premise that inhumane life-extending treatment should be precluded as a matter of social policy. When, however, life can be extended without obvious inhumanity, society must allow extension if the person has requested it by advance directive or, in the absence of a directive, if family members request it.

Because the debate over quality of life and sanctity of life is so important to society and because many engaged in the debate offer degrees of significant insight, we ought not to allow this matter to be subsumed under the more scientific-sounding term, medical futility. As I have contended throughout this book, a culture shaped by the values of cognition and capitalist-productivity will invariably tend to define quality of life in terms that discriminate against those who are infirm of mind. I have argued for a serious implementation of a quality-of-life ethic that does not so discriminate but does discourage a great deal of invasive medical treatment based on the shared value of humaneness, that is, the prohibition against causing suffering. I applied this value to people with dementia and think it applicable to other conditions of severe mental impairment, such as severe retardation.

Finally, I wish to reemphasize that a quality-of-life ethic that goes beyond humaneness is generally a self-fulfilling prophecy. Instead of comparing people with severe dementia with dogs, as does Brock, better to focus on the use of companion animals in dementia care to enhance emotional and relational quality of life. Research indicates that pet-facilitated programs in nursing homes are beneficial: pets "foster sociability, animate the withdrawn, enhance morale, fulfil needs to nurture and be nurtured, reduce reliance on psychotropic medication, and provide significant forms of sensory stimulation" (Savishinsky, 1992, p. 1325). It is amazing how much a puppy will stimulate and elicit positive emotional reaction from people with dementia who might otherwise seem too incapacitated to respond. If we believe that people with dementia can have an enhanced quality of life, then we will act on that belief.

EIGHT

✜ Dementia, Assisted Suicide, and Euthanasia

Alzheimer disease and other irreversible neurodegenerative diseases are on the cutting edge of a national and international debate over physician-assisted suicide and euthanasia. The policies that emerge from this debate will have monumental significance for people with dementia and for social attitudes toward the arduous task of providing care when preemptive death is cheaper and easier. What is cheap and easy, however, may not be best.

Before entering this debate, clarification of terms is essential. Rather than confuse the debate with the terms "active" and "passive" euthanasia, which seem to suggest two variations of what is essentially the same thing, I prefer to speak of four distinct categories of action: refusal of treatment, withdrawal of treatment, assisted suicide, and euthanasia. Refusal of any and all medical treatment is a moral and legal right for all competent Americans of age and is now increasingly sanctioned for the mature adolescent. Treatment withdrawal is no longer controversial when requested by the patient or surrogates in the context of terminal illness, and I consider irreversible dementias to be terminal even if not imminently so. Assisted suicide, however, is controversial, not just because it is death from other than the underlying disease process, but because it involves another person in the act of self-killing. Voters in Oregon, however, approved assisted suicide in November of 1994, a referendum that will doubtless be reviewed by the courts before implementation. Finally, I reserve the word "euthanasia" narrowly for those cases where death is caused by one human being ending the life of another by an act of physical impingement, whether through a lethal injection of poison, asphyxiation, or some like method.

To make these distinctions more clear, consider the case of the neonatologist who, after consulting with the parents of a premature infant with little or no hope of long-term survival, removed the mechanical respirator. This was a legally acceptable instance of treatment withdrawal, consistent with the fact that most Americans who die in hospitals do so after life-extending technologies have been experimented with, are found nonbeneficial medically or in the light of patient values, and removed. But when the infant continued to breathe independently, the physician allegedly placed a hand over the infant's trachea and leaned down until it suffocated. This second act was euthanasia, is legally unacceptable, and resulted in a grand jury investigation.

While requests for assisted suicide that result from untreated pain and inadequate psychosocial support in cases of a disease such as cancer can be deflected by hospice care, what of requests by people with a diagnosis of progressive dementia that will ultimately lead to severe loss of memory? Reports consistently indicate that in the Netherlands, where assisted suicide and mercy killing are de facto accepted, about 10 percent of requests come from patients with chronic degenerative neurological disorders (de Wachter, 1992). Margaret P. Battin writes of progressive dementia: "This is the condition the Dutch call *entluistering*, the 'effacement' or complete eclipse of human personality, and for the Dutch, *entluistering* rather than pain is a primary reason for choices of [active] euthanasia" (Battin, 1992, p. 123).

In 1990 the Michigan pathologist Jack Kevorkian assisted Janet Adkins, a 54-year-old member of the Hemlock Society diagnosed with probable AD, in suicide. Happily married with three grown sons and intellectually very active, she was horrified by the prospects of decline. One year after diagnosis, she perceived the "first symptoms" of dementia; assisted suicide at the hands of Kevorkian followed soon thereafter. Her sons and husband appear to have respected her decision to die. While few except Kevorkian would consider such an early preemptive suicide justifiable, there are those in our society who would prefer such surcease suicide rather than endure the more severe stages of dementia.

This preference is understandable. But were such preferences legally permitted and widely implemented, what would be the impact on the development of dementia care both in our communities and in long-term care institutions? Would society be willing to invest in special care units (SCUs) and caregiver training when preemptive suicide is virtually cost free? In this chapter, I will address this impact under the rubric of the "incompatibility thesis." I will then turn to other reasons, mostly cultural, as to why assisted suicide is a socially damaging response to dementia. I conclude with a discussion of dementia and hope.

The Incompatibility Hypothesis

Even if popular referendums for assisted suicide and euthanasia are eventually passed in some states in the United States, as has already occurred in Oregon, implementation should be delayed until nationwide hospice and long-term care systems for people with dementia are developed. Otherwise, these practices are likely to obviate said development. This "incompatibility hypothesis" has received insufficient attention in recent debates about assisted suicide and euthanasia—most of which are focused on individual rights, rather than on implications for the health care system. Without the full development of affordable long-term care systems in the United States, assisted suicide would be a forced default option for people with the diagnosis of dementia rather than a choice between real alternatives.

I propose to identify this concern, which has been an undercurrent in recent debate, with the term "incompatibility hypothesis"; that is, in a health care system that fails to provide adequate comfort care for the dying or long-term care for the dependent, legalization of assisted suicide and voluntary euthanasia is likely to prove incompatible with the development of such care.

Regarding comfort care, a recent study indicates that despite published guidelines for pain management, many patients with cancer have considerable pain and receive seriously inadequate analgesia (Cleeland et al., 1994). Comfort for the dying has not been a high educational or institutional priority in the United States (Callahan, 1993). Because our health care system is designed more to rescue people from death than to make dying less burdensome, the development of care for those who are dying is not a highly esteemed goal.

With regard to AD, it is important to develop more SCUs in nursing homes shaped by a commitment to the principle that something can be done for the person with dementia, even though a cure is not possible. Instead of the pervasive sense of hopelessness that can be present in nursing homes, there must be education in and commitment to the improvement of functioning and quality of life for people with dementia. "Excess disability," or "functional impairment that is greater than is warranted by an individual's disease or condition," can be removed by environmental modification, stimulation, and medical care. The residual strengths of individuals can be the foundation for enhanced quality of life; for example, people with dementia often recall how to perform tasks from earlier in their lives. It can be assumed that the behavior of people with dementia represents understandable feeling and needs that, if responded to, may be resolved without resorting to psychotropic medications or physical restraints. Yet according to recent data, only about 10 percent of nursing homes have SCUs for people with dementia (Maslow, 1994).

The costs of developing SCUs, of training home caregivers in the principles of affirmative dementia care, and of providing respite services and community programs are considerable. It is easy to imagine that the incentive to invest in dementia care will be undercut by a culture in which "final exit" is the expected alternative to societal responsibilities (Holmes et al., 1994).

In summary, my hypothesis is this: If assisted suicide or voluntary euthanasia are implemented before a fully adequate care system, the following are incurred: *(a)* diverting funds from hospice and dementia care; *(b)* undermining the training of physicians, nurses, and others for hospice and dementia; and *(c)* diminishing research in palliation or better long-term care design.

Current Discussion of Incompatibility

Others have indicated concerns akin to mine, but only in the context of hospice care. Albert R. Jonsen, a critic of assisted suicide, asks, "If pain can be ended by the death of the patient, why persist in the careful titration of medicine and emotional support that relieves pain and, at the same time, supports life" (Jonsen, 1991)? Although others seem to be concerned with the incompatibility hypothesis, they continue to defend assisted suicide. For example, Timothy E. Quill et al. fleetingly mention concern about better palliation and comfort care, acknowledge that such care in almost all cases results in a tolerable death, but then defend assisted suicide so long as the alternatives have "at least been considered" (Quill, Cassel, and Meier, 1992). The authors allude to the possibility that assisted suicide will become a substitute for comprehensive comfort care.

In a later set of regulations proposed for physician-assisted suicide, of which Quill is a coauthor, a correction is at last made: "As a treatment of last resort, physician-assisted death becomes a legitimate option only after standard measures for comfort care have been found unsatisfactory by competent patients in the context of their own situation and values" (Miller et al., 1994, p. 119). These proposed regulations go so far as to allow certified palliative-care consultants the authority to override agreements by physicians and patients to undertake assisted-suicide. The regulations indicate that this would be a spur to education in and implementation of comfort care.

Importantly, these regulations specifically argue that if terminally ill patients are allowed the option of assisted suicide and euthanasia, then so also must people with neurodegenerative diseases such as multiple sclerosis, lest they be discriminated against. This category would clearly include progressive dementias. The person with dementia is not concerned with physical pain but with the anxiety of mental deterioration. The problem of dementia is that of mental suffering in the form of anxiety and grief as memory fades; it is the problem of justified fear of loss of self and therefore of self-control.

Dan W. Brock discusses incompatibility but does not consider it a major obstacle to assisted suicide or euthanasia. Especially in a time when cost control seems essential to the future of health care and when rationing is under discussion, he writes that some foresee legalization of euthanasia as weakening society's financial commitment to "provide optimal care for dying patients" (Brock, 1993). In response, Brock says, "We should do nothing to weaken" patients' access to adequate care and services.

It can be argued that incompatibility is not applicable to health care matters. For example, acceptance of the right to withdraw or withhold life-sustaining therapy did not preclude the development of new forms of such therapy; indeed, these technologies continue to develop at a fast pace, and resources are invested in them. Therefore, the argument runs, it is unlikely that legalization of assisted suicide and euthanasia will hamper development of other options. Perhaps the availability of assisted suicide and euthanasia would even spur opponents of these practices to mobilize resources and develop state-of-the-art hospice and long-term care systems for people with dementia.

Although this hypothesis seems reasonable in the abstract, such mobilization may not garner much support in hard economic times because assisted suicide and mercy killing obviously save money. A more cautious approach would be to mandate the development of good care facilities before the quicker and cheaper options are in place. An even more cautious approach would require a trial of palliation and comfort care before acceding to any patient's wish to die (Miller et al., 1994). If such an approach is successful, many patients will lose interest in assisted suicide or euthanasia; if hospice or long-term care were prerequisites for suicide or euthanasia, they would be indirectly supported even by those patients who still wished to die.

In a country in which everyone is provided with the option of good comfort and dementia, the incompatibility hypothesis would be irrelevant. Because care in the United States for those dying painfully and for people with dementia leaves much to be desired, the fact that most people in the hospice field take the incompatibility hypothesis seriously should be closely examined.

Hospice workers' opposition to assisted suicide may be influenced by a somewhat dogmatic orthodoxy that palliation and comfort care are the best roads to death, and a sense of heresy when central dogma is contradicted. This is an orthodoxy that may change in the future. It is also logical to assume that hospice workers, whose vocation is most threatened by suicide, would be deeply concerned about incompatibility. Skepticism aside, however, hospice workers present cogent empirical, experiential, and ethical reasons for their opposition to assisted suicide and mercy killing.

Robert J. Miller writes, "The basic principles of modern pain control have been developed out of the hospice experience" (Miller, 1992). He describes the hospice movement's strong commitment to patient autonomy, which includes choices regarding the removal of artificial nutrition and hydration as well as any and all other treatments unrelated to palliation. Miller's survey of hospice staff (including nurses, physicians, administrators, social workers, and volunteers) indicates that only 5 percent favor assisted suicide, and only 1.5 percent favor mercy killing; 55 to 65 percent of respondents in public opinion surveys favor these options. Miller observes: "Those most in a position to see the daily degree of suffering of the dying, and most in a position to act on it (the nurses and doctors) were the least likely to agree to perform such acts." The major reason for this opposition was that it would "divert attention away from efforts to provide optimal palliation and more appropriate and compassionate terminal care."

Quill, long a hospice physician, would be among those advocating assisted suicide for the small but significant number of patients who cannot or will not be helped by even the best comfort care. He is a powerful proponent of hospice care, laments the lack of financial support for it, and is critical of medical education for giving insufficient attention palliative treatment. Yet his notion of death with "dignity" includes intellectual dignity as well as freedom from physical pain. This opens the door for him to justify assisted suicide in the case of a person with AIDS who fears AIDS-related dementia (1993). While Quill's opinion is shared by only a minority of hospice workers, it may have considerable influence in changing attitudes among them.

The current orthodox view among hospice physicians has recently been examined by David Cundiff (Cundiff, 1992). Cundiff contrasts assisted suicide with the routine practices of treatment refusal or withdrawal upon request. According to polls of cancer specialists, requests for assisted suicide are very uncommon. Those requests that Cundiff has heard stem from poor pain control and/or inadequate psychosocial support. Those who make requests "almost always change their minds once their physical symptoms are controlled and they are placed in a caring, supportive, hospice environment." Cundiff's thesis is that "vastly improved hospice training for health care professionals, along with better quality and greater availability of hospice services can render the issues of euthanasia and assisted suicide essentially moot."

Truog et al. (1992), on the other hand, describe several cases in which nonlethal use of barbiturates was indicated in the case of terminally ill patients whose pain could not be controlled. Sedation, in the form of a barbiturate-induced coma, is advocated as a reasonable approach that stops short of killing.

Cundiff's arguments are consistent with Miller's conclusions that "Most studies of the final days of dying patients in hospice, however, have shown that patients die peacefully and only the exceptional case requires sedation." Experienced clinicians, Miller argues, find that "unmanageable patients" are "too rare to consider changing traditional medical practice." Of course, even knowing that they represent only 2 to 5 percent of cases is no consolation to those individuals who are beyond the powers of palliative care.

Dementia Suicide

While pain is largely controllable in the hospice context for cancer patients and others, what of those who face the deep loss of memory? The incompatibility hypothesis would be relevant in such cases if assisted suicide and euthanasia were legally permitted before good AD care programs were developed to enable patients to better adapt to their incapacities. Why invest in dementia care research, training, and facilities when assisted suicide or mercy killing are already available and much cheaper?

The incompatibility hypothesis can be extended beyond dementia care to the care of the aged in general. For example, Derek Humphrey of the National Hemlock Society suggests that elderly people are crying out for death. He argues that old age is "sufficient cause to give up," even without unbearable suffering. He presents the case of an 85-year-old, recently widowed member of the Hemlock Society who took an overdose of medication and died: "There was no terminal illness, but her horror of having a stroke and spending her final years in the hospital was unbearable now that her beloved husband was gone and her children grown and scattered" (Humphrey, 1992). Her neighbor called Humphrey complaining that just the previous day this woman was walking happily in the garden. Humphrey reminded the caller that the woman was a "regular attender of Hemlock conferences for years and had clearly thought the matter through very thoroughly." At no point does Humphrey consider the possibility that improved social supports might provide an alternative to preemptive suicide among elderly people.

If assisted suicide and mercy killing were to become the way of death for the elderly, a practice defended in C. G. Prado's book on "preemptive suicide in advanced age," it is difficult to imagine continuing social commitment to institutions that enhance the quality of life for those who grow aged (Prado, 1990). In a society that some consider ageist and in which the traditional teaching functions of the elderly have all but disappeared, it is regretfully easy for preemptive suicide to become the expected choice.

The incompatibility hypothesis can be considered independently of this debate, although it begs the question. The narrow hypothesis is: If hospice and long-term care were fully developed and available nationwide, assisted suicide and euthanasia might not be chosen by many patients or people with dementia; therefore, development should occur before such practices are introduced.

Otherwise, suicide, assisted suicide, and euthanasia become the answers to terminal or dementing illness. Momentum to expend resources in areas such as long-term care and hospice slows dramatically. While this scenario is only conjectural, one should remember the old Jewish aphorism, "Start worrying. Letter to follow."

It is important to note the relationship between the appeal of assisted suicide for dementia patients and the inadequacy of living will laws and state policies. According to Henry R. Glick, current laws and policies in the United States tend to be restrictive both by limiting their scope to terminal illness, often narrowly defined, and by limiting the kinds of treatment that can be withdrawn (Glick, 1992). While some laws deal with patients in the persistent vegetative state, dementia is ignored. Moreover, the sanctions on doctors and hospitals for failing to comply with living wills are weak. Glick advocates the removal of many of the current restrictions on treatment withdrawal. Much of the societal support for assisted suicide and mercy killing is a reaction to restrictive laws in the area of treatment refusal and withdrawal. Allowing assisted suicide and mercy killing may undermine efforts to correct these laws.

There is a choice in the American future between *(a)* the status quo health care system, in which dementia care is inadequately supported and receives relatively little attention in medical education; *(b)* a system of medicalized killing and geronticide that is the inevitable product of this inattention; and *(c)* a system that makes dementia care an essential raison d'etre. If the third option is a compelling one, it may be incompatible with assisted suicide and mercy killing, since these remove the needy individuals who collectively create the social pressure for this raison d'etre.

Spilling Over: The Culture of Thanatos

Humphrey, in his controversial book *Final Exit,* proposes that society accept assisted suicide and euthanasia not just for the terminally ill, but also for *(a)* the spouse whose loved one is dying and wishes to "go together"; *(b)* those with spinal chord injuries; and *(c)* those who are just getting old

(1991). While I disagree with Humphrey, I appreciate his honesty in acknowledging that assisted suicide would be difficult to limit to the context of terminal illness. The spillover of this practice from terminal care to other regions of human experience that challenge the will to live is unavoidable.

Since guidelines were established in 1984, the Netherlands has permitted de facto assisted suicide and euthanasia, although they have limited this practice to the terminally ill, including people with progressive dementias. Since December 1993, exclusion of physicians from criminal prosecution for assisted suicide and euthanasia has been established in law, according to which the patient must be suffering unbearably, be in the terminal phase of illness, and have expressed the will to die, more than once. In June 1994, the Dutch Supreme Court went further. It ruled that Dr. Boudewijn Chabot could not be prosecuted for assisting in the suicide of a 50-year-old woman who was suffering after the deaths of her two sons. Chabot's patient could not cope with life, and he decided, after seeing her for twenty-four hours total, that her wish to die was genuine. Subsequently, "He provided her with the lethal preparation, which she drank in his presence and that of a friend and her general practitioner. Chabot then reported the case to judicial authorities, as required by law" (Spanjer, 1994, p. 1630). The Supreme Court judgment clarified that now mental suffering is a legally acceptable reason for assisted suicide.

Now if assisted suicide is an acceptable response to mental suffering (applicable to people who are competent), then it is viable for most of us, since few people get through life without considerable grief. Instead of pursuing standard psychiatric treatment through "grief analysis," the solution in the Netherlands is to remove the griever and thereby the grief. The problems of an existential nature that challenge the character of every man and woman no longer must be resolved creatively; they are cause for a "final exit" instead.

It is my view that assisted suicide in the context of terminal illness is *not* best understood purely in terms of an individual's right to die. Rather, it must be placed in a communitarian context in which responsibilities for the common good as well as rights have moral importance. People with severe incurable diseases have responsibilities to maintain the general cultural prohibition against suicide as a routine response to life's inevitable challenges. The spillover from terminal care into other areas of human experience is, if the Netherlands is our example, almost inevitable.

It is this notion of spillover that underlies the current legal restrictions on assisted suicide in the United States and in all European nations other than the Netherlands. Perhaps, taken in pure isolation, some cases of assisted suicide or euthanasia are morally tolerable. But in the United States, those who engage in such actions must face a jury and in most but not all instances are going to receive merciful judgment.

Physicians have long shortened the lives of the dying with palliative treatments (e.g., morphine) intended only to prevent suffering. The doctrine of "double effect" indicates that so long as the intention is to prevent suffering and the life shortening is an unintended although foreseeable side effect, no moral error is committed. This doctrine can obviously be debated, for how can the foreseeable shortening of life not be directly intended unless the moral agent is bifurcated? Nevertheless, the doctrine serves society well by allowing action that approximates euthanasia to be carried out in the privacy of the doctor-patient relationship and under the auspices of control of suffering rather than removal of the sufferer.

To condone by law and policy the removal of the sufferer is to sanction actions that cannot be narrowly contained and circumscribed. We invite culture in which courage, endurance, hope, love, and creativity in the face of the burdens of living are set aside and replaced by feeble purpose, low ideals, fear of discomfort, and the inability to go through disappointment without losing heart. For those who doubt this, the recent development in the Netherlands provides a case in point.

Classically, the major arguments against suicide have been that (a) it is an arrogant usurpation of the authority of God who both giveth and taketh away life; (b) it shows lack of faith in creative resolutions of relational and other difficulties; (c) it has the ripple effect of encouraging others to follow suit; and (d) it is contrary to true human nature and therefore never an authentic desire. The first and fourth of these arguments can be easily objected to. Appeal to divine command does not carry much rational weight, and people who wish to die are not always irrational and in violation of human nature. The second and third, however, have merit, especially in a time of social anomie and loss of meaning.

The spillover of assisted suicide and euthanasia would of course at first be limited to cases of voluntary self-destruction. But as self-destruction becomes the cultural expectation, it can be tyrannical even if freely chosen. Those who wish to live on would receive the powerful look of opprobrium, as though they are merely wasting resources. Might it not become the standard expectation that the old extinguish themselves?

It is here that I assert the sanctity of life. As Karl Barth wrote: "A man who is not, or is no longer, capable of work, of earning, of enjoyment and even perhaps of communication, is not for this reason unfit to live, least of all because he cannot render to the existence of the state any notable or active contribution, but can only directly or indirectly burden it. The value of this kind of life is God's secret" (Barth, 1961, p. 423). Assisted suicide and euthanasia become excuses for society to no longer manifest the strength to carry its weak and weakest members, and this is a sign of moral collapse. Instead of a culture of *cura* (care) we will have the culture of *thanatos* (death). The involvement of the medical profession in assisted suicide and suicide would further erode respect for life and confuse the identity of the physician.

The notion of spillover suggests that the permission for assisted suicide and euthanasia is difficult to contain within the narrow context of care for the terminally ill. But my misgivings go even further to what the sociologist Emil Durkheim described as obligatory altruistic suicide in his classic 1897 study *Suicide* (Durkheim, 1952; Berrios and Mohanna, 1990). Such suicide is not obligatory by law, but by cultural expectation; that is, it comes to be viewed as selfish to live.

My argument here is that while the isolated individual act of assisted suicide might be justifiable, when viewed in the context of the common good, it must be rejected because of repercussions. Suicide, instead of being viewed as wrong or at best as morally ambiguous, would come to be viewed as an act of justice intended to remove undue burdens on families and society. What would initially be a choice made by the few would become an obligation for the many. The counterargument is that appeals to a hypothetical public good must be made with great care and circumspection; that is, just because assisted suicide and euthanasia are available does not mean that everyone will feel obliged to request them (Helme, 1993).

I wish to conclude this section by indicating that contrary to those who champion the cause of suicide, it is not as attractive an option as they suggest. For example, Humphrey, in *Final Exit*, condones "going together." He gives the case of the perfectly healthy 55-year-old wife of 77-year-old novelist Arthur Koestler who drank poison with her terminally ill husband (1991). Yet gerontologist Robert Kastenbaum summarizes a series of empirical studies indicating that suicide is not a dominant theme among elderly men and women experiencing terminal illness (1992). Those who survive the challenges of life and reach old age are a tough lot with "relatively low orientation toward self-destruction." Anger, despair, and suicidality do arise "from painful conditions of life rather than from the prospect of death." Kastenbaum presents the case of an elderly woman dying of cancer who, once given comfort and pain relief, would prefer to continue on with life. He supports preventive responses to suicidality along with wide recognition of how unusual self-destructive orientation is when life circumstances are improved through psychosocial interventions and palliation. While we are to "understand and respect" the framework that makes suicide an attractive option for some, elderly people when well cared for are not crying out for death.

Also in contrast to Humphrey, Joseph Richman is surprised by the volume of writing on assisted suicide, when it is rarely desired (1992). Richman explores the alternatives to suicide: "Recovery from the suicidal state in the elderly is based upon relationships that support a sense of worth as an individual and provide a sense of belonging and social cohesion." Richman laments "a great publicity campaign in favor of the view that suicide is a rational response to growing old." Such a campaign "discourages a life-enhancing resolution to problems in living" (p. 133). What we need, he believes, are more rights for the elderly than the mere but cheap right to die.

Dementia and Hope

This book began with an ethics of hope for people with dementia that is predicated on the possibility for quality of life despite the deepest forgetfulness. The forms of emotional and relational affirmation that constitute good dementia care were discussed; and optimism was expressed that more residual self-identity may be present than the chaos of communicative breakdown suggests.

In concluding this book, I wish to consider the moral dynamics of hope and specifically examine the role of hope in the care of people with dementia.

Contemporary medical law and ethics have achieved much for patient self-determination based on physician disclosure of information. Hope is rightly castigated as having provided justification for paternalistic lies and halftruths. At worst, wanton harms were garbed in hope. For example, Henry K. Beecher pointed to a case (example 18) in which melanoma was transplanted from a daughter to her informed mother "in the hope of gaining a little better understanding of cancer immunity and in the hope that the production of tumor antibodies might be helpful in the treatment of the cancer patient." The daughter was dead a day after the transplant; her mother died from metastatic melanoma 451 days later (Beecher, 1966).

In reaction against the paternalistic admonition to deceive in order to preserve hope, there is now the view that hope has no role in our thinking about medical ethics. Yet hope should not be entirely dismissed, for it is one major mode by which people anticipate the future; it is the human passion for the possible that makes difficult circumstances endurable. True hope is not wishful thinking or naive optimism that ignores reality. Hope is associated with courage and often is enhanced or weakened by the influence of others. By their words and actions, family members and health care professionals can be powerful modulators of hope in people with dementia.

Plato wrote that we are all filled with hope all of our lives (*Philebus* 39e), and this is generally true, although our hopes may become more realistic as we mature. Most people consider it solace that in the midst of present troubles they may still hope. Hope is such a central element of the human experience that it is creatively ensconced in mythologies and symbols from all civilizations. In Greek myth, Prometheus considers the human affliction of foreseeing the doom of death, in response to which Prometheus proclaims, "I caused blind hopes to dwell within their breasts" (l. 250). But the ancients warned that hope can easily be led astray. So Thucydides advised dependence "not so much in hope, which is strongest in perplexity, as in reason supported by the facts, which gives a surer insight into the future" (bk. 2, l. 62).

While the deceptions and harms perpetrated in the name of hope are not to be condoned, there remains something to be said for Thomas Percival's image of the physician as "minister of hope and comfort to the sick." Percival cited the Enlightenment philosopher Francis Hutcheson, "No man censures a Physician for deceiving a patient too much dejected, by expressing good hopes for him" (Percival, 1849).

For some cultural groups those who suggest that there is no hope are always wrong. For example, among Arab Muslims, "Hope helps a patient mobilize his own resources to cope with the illness, even if such hope is false by Western standards. As long as the patient has faith in Allah and his power, hope is never false" (Meleis and Jonsen, 1983). God and hope are intertwined, although this does not entail deception. We need not adopt the Islamic standard to recognize the importance of hope in the care of people with dementia.

That hope has traditionally been a value in ethics suggests that its general absence from current medical ethics literature is unacceptable, even if understandable as a reaction against strong paternalism. An exception is the writing of James Drane, who notes that "Because despair is so painful and so frequently part of the dying process, it is not too much to say that it falls within the scope of a doctor's ministrations. Each physical loss causes a certain amount of despair, and when physical disintegration slips beyond medical help, despair may be severe" (1988, p. 56).

The virtue of truthfulness requires sensitivity and subtlety because human beings are in part constituted by their hopes. Good caregivers encourage no groundless hopes, nor do they wantonly lie. But the ability to nurture hope in the context of dementia care is an essential art. Drane observes that "Despair is painful because it is the nature of human beings to hope" (p. 125).

Human beings project or throw themselves forward into the future. It is important to remember that many people with dementia are motivated and supported by nothing more or less than hope for a good and dignified death, which they plan for through specifying their wishes. Hope does not justify deception, but it demands that people with dementia have the security of knowing that the effects of their disease will be treated, that much will be done to ensure their emotional well-being as their dementia progresses, that their directives for treatment levels will be adhered to so long as no pain or suffering results, that they will be provided with opportunities to engage in meaningful activities, and that they will have the benefit of support groups.

By giving people with dementia this hope for dignified care, the appeal of assisted suicide becomes less powerful. People with dementia can also know that they need not be subjected to the exclusionary forces of a society that overvalues cognition as the defining feature of being human. Their forgetfulness, even when it becomes quite full, does not mean that they will lack the care and respect of others. There is more hope for more people with dementia in an ethos of solicitous care and enhanced quality of life than in joining the flight to suicide.

Will there be a cure for AD, the prototypical disorder for progressive and irreversible dementias? Perhaps drugs will be developed to replace neurotransmitters or to enhance the growth of brain cells. Genetic studies may unlock the mechanisms of dementia so that cures can be found. It is important to be hopeful about the horizon of cure (Khachaturian, 1992). For now, however, the hope for people with dementia rests almost entirely in the commitment of family members, professional caregivers, and society to their well-being.

⅔ References

Adamson, E. (1990). *Art as Healing.* Boston: Coventure.

Advisory Panel on Alzheimer's Disease (1991). *Third Report of the Advisory Panel on Alzheimer's Disease.* Washington, D.C.: U.S. Department of Health and Human Services.

Agich, G. J. (1993). *Autonomy and Long-Term Care.* New York: Oxford University Press.

Alemayehu, E., Molloy, D. W., Guyatt, G. H. (1991). Variability in physicians' decisions on caring for chronically ill elderly patients: an international study. *Canadian Medical Association Journal,* 144:1133–38.

Algase, D. L. (1992). A century of progress: today's strategies for responding to wandering behavior. *Journal of Gerontological Nursing,* 18 (11):28–34.

Alzheimer Society of Canada (1992). *Guidelines for Care.* Toronto: Alzheimer Society of Canada.

Annas, G. J., and Glantz, L. H. (1986). The right of elderly patients to refuse life-sustaining treatment. *Milbank Quarterly,* 64 (suppl. 2):95–162.

Appelbaum, P. S., and Grisso, T. (1988). Assessing patients' capacities to consent to treatment. *Journal of the American Medical Association,* 319:1635–38.

Arras, J. (1988). The severely demented, minimally functional patient: an ethical analysis. *Journal of the American Geriatrics Society,* 36:938–44.

Asch, A. (1989). Can aborting 'imperfect' children be immoral? In J. Arras and N. Rhoden, eds., *Ethical Issues in Modern Medicine,* pp. 317–21. Mountain View, Calif.: Mayfield Publishing.

Bagnell, P. D., and Soper, P. S., eds. (1989). *Perceptions of Aging in Literature: A Cross-Cultural Study.* New York: Greenwood Press.

Barth, K. (1961). *The Doctrine of Creation: Church Dogmatics, Vol. III, Part Four.* Edinburgh: T. & T. Clark.

Battin, M. P. (1992). Euthanasia in Alzheimer's disease? In R. H. Binstock, S. G. Post, and P. J. Whitehouse, eds., *Dementia and Aging: Ethics, Values, and Policy Choices,* pp. 118–37. Baltimore: Johns Hopkins University Press.

Beecher, H. K. (1966). Ethics and clinical research. *New England Journal of Medicine,* 274:1354–60.

Bellah, R. (1985) *Habits of the Heart.* New York: Harper Collins.

Berdyaev, N. (1937) *The Destiny of Man.* N. Duddington, trans. London: Geoffrey Bless.

Berg, J. M., Karlinsky, H., and Holland, A. J., eds. (1993). *Alzheimer Disease, Down Syndrome, and their Relationship.* New York: Oxford University Press.

Bernlef, J. (1989). *Out of Mind.* Boston: David R. Godine.

Berrios, G. E., and Mohanna, M. (1990). Durkheim and French psychiatric views on suicide during the 19th century: a conceptual history. *British Journal of Psychiatry,* 156:1–9.

Binstock, R. H., and Post, S. G., eds. (1991). *Too Old for Health Care? Controversies in Medicine, Law, Economics, and Ethics.* Baltimore: Johns Hopkins University Press.

Binstock, R. H., Post, S. G., and Whitehouse, P. J., eds. (1992). *Dementia and Aging: Ethics, Values, and Policy Choice.* Baltimore: Johns Hopkins University Press.

Birren, J. E., and Dieckmann, L. (1991). Concepts and content of quality of life in the later years: an overview. In J. E. Birren, C. R. Rowe, J. E. Lubben, and D. E. Deutchman, eds. *The Concept and Measurement of Quality of Life in the Frail Elderly,* pp. 344–60. New York: Academic Press, 1991.

Blessed, G., Tomlinson, B. E., Roth, M. (1968). The association between quantitative measures of dementia and of senile change in the grey matter of elderly subjects. *British Journal of Psychiatry,* 138:797–811.

Boller, F., Forette, F., Khachaturian, Z., Poncet, M., Christen, Y., eds. (1992). *Heterogeneity of Alzheimer's Disease.* Berlin: Springer-Verlag.

Botkin, J. R., and Alemagno, S. (1992). Carrier screening for cystic fibrosis: a pilot study of attitudes of pregnant women. *American Journal of Public Health,* 82:723–25.

Branch, L. G., and Jette, A. M. (1982). A prospective study of long-term care institutionalization among the aged. *American Journal of Public Health,* 72:1373–78.

Brandt, J., Quaid, K., Folstein, S. E., et al. (1989). Presymptomatic diagnosis of delayed-onset disease with linked DNA markers: the experience of Huntington's disease. *Journal of the American Medical Association,* 21:3108–14.

Breitner, J. C. S. (1991). Clinical genetics and genetic counseling in Alzheimer disease. *Annals of Internal Medicine,* 115:601–5.

Brinton, C. (1959). *A History of Western Morals.* New York: Harcourt, Brace and Co.

Brock, D. W. (1988). Justice and the severely demented elderly. *Journal of Medicine and Philosophy,* 13:73–99.

Brock, D. W. (1993). *Life and Death: Philosophical Essays in Biomedical Ethics.* New York: Cambridge University Press.

Brody, E. M., (1990). *Women in the Middle: Their Parent-Care Years.* New York: Springer Publishing.

Buchanan, A. E., and Brock, D. W. (1990). *Deciding for Others: The Ethics of Surrogate Decision Making.* New York: Cambridge University Press.

Buchanon, J. H. (1989). *Patient Encounters: The Experience of Disease.* Charlottesville: University of Virginia Press.

Burns, A., and Levy, R. (1993). *Clinical Diversity in Late Onset Alzheimer's Disease.* New York: Oxford University Press.

Callahan, D. (1987). *Setting Limits: Medical Goals in an Aging Society.* New York: Simon & Schuster.

Callahan, D. (1993). *The Troubled Dream of Life: Living with Mortality*. New York: Simon & Schuster.

Callahan, S. (1992). Ethics and dementia: quality of life. *Alzheimer Disease and Associated Disorders*, 6(3):138–44.

Carter, S. L. (1993). *The Culture of Disbelief: How American Law and Politics Trivialized Religious Devotion*. New York: Basic Books.

Chafetz, P. K. (1990). Structuring environments for dementia patients. In M. F. Weiner, ed., *The Dementias: Diagnosis and Management*, pp. 249–61. Washington, D.C.: American Psychiatric Press.

Chatterjee, A., Strauss, M. E., Smyth, K. A., and Whitehouse, P. J. (1992). Personality changes in Alzheimer's disease. *Archives of Neurology*, 49:486–91.

Cleeland, C. S., Gonin, R., Hatfield, A. K., Blum, R. H., Stewart, J. A., and Kishan, J. P. (1994). Pain and its treatment in outpatients with metastatic cancer. *New England Journal of Medicine*, 330:592–96.

Clifford, D. B., and Glicksman, M. (1994). AIDS dementia. In J. C. Morris, ed., *Handbook of Dementing Illnesses*, pp. 441–95. New York: Marcel Dekker.

Cohen, C., Kennedy, G., and Eisdorfer, C. (1984). Phases of change in the patient with Alzheimer's dementia: a conceptual dimension for defining health care management. *Journal of the American Geriatrics Society*, 32:11–15.

Cohen-Mansfield, J., Droge, J. A., and Billig, N. (1992). Factors influencing hospital patients' preferences in the utilization of life-sustaining treatments. *Gerontologist*, 32:89-95.

Cohen-Mansfield, J., Werner, P., Marx, M. S., and Freedman, L. (1991). Two studies of pacing in the nursing home. *Journals of Gerontology*, 46(3):M77–83.

Cook-Deegan, R. M. (1994). Ethical issues arising in the search for neurological disease genes. In N. Fujiki, D. R. J. Macer, eds. *Intractable Neurological Disorders, Human Genome Research and Society: Proceedings of the Third International Bioethics Seminar in Fukui, 19–21 November 1993*, pp. 81–92. Tokyo: Eubios Ethics Institute.

Corder, E. H., Saunders, A. M., Risch, N.J., et al. (1994). Protective effect of apolipoprotein E type 2 allele for late onset Alzheimer disease. *Nature Genetics*, 7:180–84.

Corder, E. H., Saunders, A. M., Strittmatter, W. J., et al. (1993). Gene dose of apolipoprotein E type 4 allele and the risk of Alzheimer's disease in late-onset families. *Science*, 261:921–23.

Corson, V., Quaid, K., Kasch, L., and Kazazian, H. H. (1990). Prenatal testing for Huntington disease. In B. A. Fine, ed., *Strategies in Genetic Counseling: Reproductive Genetics & New Technologies*, pp. 226–30. Washington, D.C.: March of Dimes Birth Defects Foundation.

Coughlan, P. A. (1993). *Facing Alzheimer's: Family Caregivers Speak*. New York: Ballantine Books.

Cranford, R. E. (1991). Helga Wanglie's ventilator. *Hastings Center Report*, 21 (4):23–24.

Cundiff, D. (1992). *Euthanasia Is Not the Answer: A Hospice Physician's View*. Totowa, N. J.: Humana Press.

Danis, M., Sutherland, L. I., Garrett, J. M., et al. (1991). A prospective study of advance directives for life-sustaining care. *New England Journal of Medicine,* 324:882–888.

Darling, R. (1979). *Families Against Society.* Beverly Hills, Calif.: Sage Library of Social Research.

Davis, K. L., Thal, L. J., Gamzu, E. R., et al. (1992). A double-blind, placebo-controlled multicenter study of tacrine for Alzheimer's disease. *New England Journal of Medicine,* 327:1253–59.

Davis, R. (with help from his wife, Betty). (1989). *My Journey into Alzheimer's Disease.* Wheaton, Ill.: Tyndale House Publishers.

Day, J. J., Grant, I., Atkinson, J. H., and Richman, D. D. (1992). Incidence of AIDS dementia in a two-year follow-up of AIDS and ARC patients on an initial phase II AZT placebo-controlled study: San Diego Cohort. *Journal of Neuropsychiatry and Clinical Neurosciences,* 4:15–20.

Dennis, N. (1964). *Jonathan Swift.* New York: Collier Books.

de Wachter, M. A. M. (1992). Euthanasia in the Netherlands. *Hastings Center Report,* 22(2):23–30.

Diamond, E. L., Jernigan, J. A., Moseley, R. A., Messina, V., and McKeown, R. A. (1989). Decision-making ability and advance directive preferences in nursing home patients and proxies. *Gerontologist,* 29:622–26.

Dostoyevsky, F. (1988). *The Adolescent.* In Hutterite Brethren, eds., *The Gospel in Dostoyevsky: Selections from His Works.* Ulster, N. Y.: Plow.

Drachman, D. A. (1988). Who may drive? Who may not? Who shall decide? *Annals of Neurology,* 24: 178–87.

Drachman, D. A., and Swearer, J. M. (1993). Driving and Alzheimer's disease. *Neurology,* 43:2448–56.

Drane, J. F. (1988). *Becoming a Good Doctor: The Place of Virtue and Character in Medical Ethics.* St. Louis: Sheed & Ward.

Dresser, R. (1994). Missing persons: legal perceptions of incompetent patients. *Rutgers Law Review,* 46:609–719.

Drickamer, M. A., and Lachs, M. S. (1992). Should patients with Alzheimer's disease be told their diagnosis? *New England Journal of Medicine,* 326:947–51.

Durkheim, E. (1952). *Suicide: A Study in Sociology.* London: Routledge & Kegan Paul.

Dworkin, G. (1976). Autonomy and behavior control. *Hastings Center Report,* 6(1): 23–28.

Dworkin, R. (1993). *Life's Dominion: An Argument About Abortion, Euthanasia, and Individual Freedom.* New York: Vintage.

Englehardt, H. T. (1986). *The Foundations of Bioethics.* New York: Oxford University Press.

English, J. (1979). What do grown children owe their parents? In O. O'Neill and W. Ruddick, eds., *Having Children: Philosophical and Legal Reflections on Parenthood,* pp. 351–56. New York: Oxford University Press.

Evans, D. A., Funkenstein, H. H., Albert, M. S., et al. (1989). Prevalence of Alzheimer's disease in a community population of older persons: higher than previously reported. *Journal of the American Medical Association,* 262:2551–56.

Evans, L., and Strumpf, N. (1989). Tying down the elderly: a review of the literature on physical restraint. *Journal of the American Geriatrics Society,* 37:65–74.

Faden, R. A., Chwalow, J., Quaid, K., Chase, G. A., Lopes, C., Leonard, C. O., and Holtzman, N. A. (1987). Prenatal screening and pregnant women's attitudes toward the abortion of defective fetuses. *American Journal of Public Health* 77:288–90.

Farlow, M., Gracon, S. I., Hershey, L.A., et al. (1992). A controlled trial of tacrine in Alzheimer's disease. *Journal of the American Medical Association,* 268: 2523–29.

Feil, N. (1993). *The Validation Breakthrough: Simple Techniques for Communicating with People with "Alzheimer's-Type Dementia."* Baltimore: Health Professions Press.

Fiedler, L. A. (1985). The tyranny of the normal. In T. H. Murray and A. L. Caplan, eds., *Which Babies Shall Live? Humanistic Dimensions of the Care of Imperiled Newborns,* pp. 151–59. Clifton, N.J.: Humana Press.

Firlik, A. D. (1991). Margo's logo. *Journal of the American Medical Association,* 265:201.

Fitten, L. J., Morley, J. E., Gross, P. L., Petry, S. D., Cole, K. D. (1989). Depression: UCLA geriatric grand rounds. *Journal of the American Geriatrics Society,* 37:459–72.

Flack, H. E., and Pellegrino, E. D., eds. (1992). *African-American Perspectives on Biomedical Ethics.* Washington, D.C.: Georgetown University Press.

Fletcher, J. F. (1975). Four indicators of personhood—the enquiry matures. *Hastings Center Report,* 4 (December):4–7.

Foley, J. M. (1992). The experience of dementia. In R. H. Binstock, S. G. Post, and P. J. Whitehouse, eds., *Dementia and Aging: Ethics, Values, and Policy Choices,* pp. 30–43. Baltimore: Johns Hopkins University Press.

Foley, J. M. (1993). Marginal to useless medications. *Centerviews,* 7(2):1 and 4.

Foley, J. M., and Post, S. G. (1994). Ethical issues in dementia. In J. C. Morris, ed., *Handbook of Dementing Illnesses,* pp. 3–22. New York: Marcel Dekker.

Ford, A. B., Roy, A. W., Haug, M. R., Folmar, S. J., and Jones P. K. (1991). Impaired and disabled elderly in the community. *American Journal of Public Health,* 81:1207–9.

Foucault, M. (1965). *Madness and Civilization: A History of Insanity in the Age of Reason.* R. Howard, trans. New York: Vintage Books.

Fox, P. (1989). From senility to Alzheimer's disease: the rise of the Alzheimer's disease movement. *Milbank Quarterly,* 67:58–102.

Friedland, R. P., Koss, E., Haxby, J. V., Grady, C. L., Luxenberg, J., Schapiro, M. B., and Kaye, J. (1988). Alzheimer disease: clinical and biological heterogeneity. *Annals of Internal Medicine,* 109:298–311.

Gilley, D. W., Wilson, R. S., Bennett, D. A., Stebbins, G. T., Bernard, B. A., Whalen,

M. E., and Fox, J. H. (1991). Cessation of driving and unsafe motor vehicle operation by dementia patients. *Archives of Internal Medicine,* 151:941–46.

Gilmore, C. G., Whitehouse, P. J., and Wykle, M. L. (1989). *Memory, Aging, and Dementia: Theory, Assessment, and Treatment.* New York: Springer Publishing.

Glick, H. R. (1992). *The Right to Die: Policy Innovation and Its Consequences.* New York: Columbia University Press.

Groate, A., Chartier-Harlin, M., Mullan, M., et al. (1991). Segregation of a missense mutation in the amyloid precursor protein gene with familial Alzheimer's disease. *Nature,* 349:704–6.

Gustafson, J. M. (1981). Mongolism, parental desires, and the right to life. In T. A. Shannon, ed., *Bioethics: Basic Writings on the Key Ethical Questions That Surround the Major, Modern Biological Possibilities and Problems,* pp. 129–55. Ramsey, N. J.: Paulist Press.

Gwyther, L. P., and Blazer, D. G. (1984). Family therapy and the dementia patient. *American Family Physician,* 29 (5):149–56.

Habermas, J. (1990). *Moral Consciousness and Communicative Action.* Cambridge, Mass.: MIT Press.

Habermas, J. (1993). *Justification and Application: Remarks on Discourse Ethics.* Cambridge, Mass.: MIT Press.

Hall, E. W. (1961). *Our Knowledge of Fact and Values.* Chapel Hill: University of North Carolina Press.

Hauerwas, S. (1986). *Suffering Presence: Theological Reflections on Medicine, the Church, and the Mentally Handicapped.* Notre Dame: University of Notre Dame Press.

Hauerwas, S. (1990). *Naming the Silences: God, Medicine, and the Problem of Suffering.* Grand Rapids, Mich.: Wm. B. Eerdmans.

Hazo, R. (1967). *The Idea of Love.* New York: Frederick A. Praeger.

Hellen R. (1992). *Alzheimer's Disease: Activity-Focused Care.* Boston: Andover Medical Publishers.

Helme, T. (1993). "A special defence": a psychiatric approach to formalising euthanasia. *British Journal of Psychiatry,* 163:456–66.

Heston, L. L., Mastri, A. R., Anderson, V. E., and White, J. (1981). Dementia of the Alzheimer's type: clinical genetics, natural history, and associated conditions. *Archives of General Psychiatry,* 38:1085–90.

Hoche, A. (1992). Essay two: medical explanation. In K. Binding and A. Hoche, *Permitting the Destruction of Unworthy Life,* pp. 255–65. Reprinted verbatim, *Issues in Law and Medicine,* 8 (2):231–65.

Holmes, D., Lindeman, D., Ory, M., and Teresi, J. (1994). Measurement of service units and costs of care for persons with dementia in special care units. *Alzheimer Disease and Associated Disorders: An International Journal,* 8 (suppl. 1):328-40.

Howell, M. (1984). Caretakers' views on responsibilities for the care of the demented elderly. *Journal of the American Geriatrics Society,* 32 (9):657–60.

Humphrey, D. (1991). *Final Exit: The Practicalities of Self-Deliverance and Assisted Suicide for the Dying.* Eugene, Ore.: Hemlock Society.

Humphrey, D. (1992). Rational suicide among the elderly. In A. A. Leenaars, R. W. Maris, J. L. McIntosh, and J. Richman, eds., *Suicide and the Older Adult*, pp. 125–29. New York: Guilford Press.

Hunt, L., Morris, J. C., Edwards, E., and Wilson, B. S. (1993). Driving performance in persons with mild senile dementia of the Alzheimer type. *Journal of the American Geriatrics Society*, 41:747–53.

Huppert, F. A., Brayne, C., and O'Connor, D. W., eds. (1994). *Dementia and Normal Aging*. New York: Cambridge University Press.

Ingelfinger, F. J. (1980). Arrogance. *New England Journal of Medicine*, 303:1507-11.

Institute of Medicine (1986). *Improving the Quality of Care in Nursing Homes*. Washington, D. C.: National Academy Press.

Jedlicka-Kohler, I., Gotz, M., and Eichler, I. (1994). Utilization of prenatal diagnosis for cystic fibrosis over the past seven years. *Pediatrics*, 94:13–16.

Johnson, S. H. (1990). The fear of liability and the use of restraints in nursing homes. *Law, Medicine and Health Care: Law and Aging*, 18(3):263–73.

Jonsen, A. R. (1991). Reflection. In R. H. Hamel, ed., *Active Euthanasia, Religion, and the Public Debate*, pp. 100–105. Chicago: Park Ridge Center.

Kane, R. A. (1990). Everyday life in nursing homes: the "way things are." In R. A. Kane and A. L. Caplan, eds., *Everyday Ethics: Resolving Dilemmas in Nursing Homes*, pp. 3–20. New York: Springer Publishing.

Karjala, D. S. (1992). A legal research agenda for the human genome initiative. *Jurimetrics: Journal of Law, Science, and Technology*, 32:168.

Karlinsky, H., Lennox, A., and Rossor, M., eds. (1994). *Alzheimer Disease and Genetic Testing: Alzheimer Disease and Associated Disorders* 8 (no. 2).

Karlinsky, H., Madrick, E., Ridgley, J., et al. (1991). A family with multiple instances of definite, probable and possible early-onset Alzheimer's disease. *British Journal of Psychiatry*, 159:524–30.

Karlinsky, H., Vaula, G., Haines, J. L., et al. (1992). Molecular and prospective phenotypic characterization of a pedigree with familial Alzheimer's disease and a missense mutation in codon 717 of the beta-amyloid precursor protein gene. *Neurology*, 42:1445–53.

Kastenbaum, R. (1992). Death, suicide, and the older adult. In A. A. Leenaars, R. W. Maris, J. L. McIntosh, and J. Richman, eds., *Suicide and the Older Adult*, pp. 1–14. New York: Guilford Press.

Katz, J. (1972). *Experimentation with Human Beings*. New York: Russell Sage Foundation.

Katzman, R. (1976). The prevalence and malignancy of Alzheimer disease. *Archives of Neurology*, 33:217–18.

Katzman, R., and Saitoh, T. (1991). Advances in Alzheimer's disease. *FASEB Journal*, 5:278–86.

Kayser-Jones, J. (1990). The use of nasogastric feeding tubes in nursing homes: patients, family and health care provider perspectives. *Gerontologist*, 30: 469–79.

Kelsey, M. T. (1973). *Psychology, Medicine & Christian Healing*. San Francisco: Harper & Row.

Keniston, K. (1977). *All Our Children: The American Family Under Pressure*. New York: Harcourt Brace Jovanovich.

Khachaturian, Z. S. (1992). An overview of critical issues in developing treatments for Alzheimer's disease. *International Psychogeriatrics*, 4(supp. 1):131–35.

Kitwood, T. (1993). Towards a theory of dementia care: the interpersonal process. *Ageing and Society*, 13:51–67.

Kitwood, T., and Bredin, K. (1992). Towards a theory of dementia care: personhood and well-being. *Ageing and Society*, 12:269–87.

Klerman, G. (1975). Behavior control and the limits of reform—the use of new technologies in total institutions. *Hastings Center Report*, 5(4):40–45.

Lakoff, G., and Johnson, M. (1980). *Metaphors We Live By*. Chicago: University of Chicago Press.

Lecky, W. E. H. (1955). *History of European Morals from Augustus to Charlemagne*. New York: George Braziller.

Levine, R. J. (1986). *Ethics and Regulation of Clinical Research*. Baltimore-Munich: Urban & Schwarzenberg.

Lidz, C. W., Fischer, L., and Arnold, R. M. (1992). *The Erosion of Autonomy in Long-Term Care*. New York: Oxford University Press.

Light, E., and Lebowitz, B. D., eds. (1989). *Alzheimer's Disease Treatment and Family Stress: Directions for Research*, pp. 322–39. Rockville, Md.: U.S. Department of Health and Human Services.

Lipkowitz, R. (1988). Services for Alzheimer patients and their families. In M. K. Aronson, ed., *Understanding Alzheimer's Disease*, pp. 198–226. New York: Charles Scribner's Sons.

Lo, B. (1990). Assessing decision-making capacity. *Law, Medicine and Health Care: Law and Aging*, 18(3):193–201.

Loewry, E. H. (1987). Decisions in the mentally impaired: limiting but not abandoning treatment. *New England Journal of Medicine*, 317:1465–69.

Lomas, J. (1986). The consensus process and evidence dissemination. *Canadian Medical Association Journal*, 134:1340–41.

Lomas, J., and Jacoby, I. (1985). The town meeting for technology: the maturation of consensus conferences. *Journal of the American Medical Association*, 254:1068–72.

Lowenberg, K., and Waggoner, R. (1934). Familial organic psychosis (Alzheimer's type). *Archives of Neurology*, 31:737–54.

Lucas, E. T. (1991). *Elder Abuse and Its Recognition Among Health Service Professionals*. New York: Garland.

Lynn, J. (1988). Conflicts of interest in medical decision making. *Journal of the American Geriatrics Society*, 36:945–50.

Mace, N. L. (1990). The management of problem behaviors. In N. L. Mace, ed., *Dementia Care: Patient, Family, and Community*, pp. 74–112. Baltimore: Johns Hopkins University Press.

Mace, N. L., and Rabins, P. V. (1991). *The 36-Hour Day.* Baltimore: Johns Hopkins University Press.

Marcel, G. (1956). *The Philosophy of Existentialism,* M. Harari, trans. Secaucus, N.J.: Citadel Press.

Martin, R. J., and Post, S. G. (1992). Human dignity, dementia, and the moral basis of caregiving. In R. H. Binstock, S. G. Post, and P. J. Whitehouse, eds., *Dementia and Aging: Ethics, Values, and Policy Choices,* pp. 55–68. Baltimore: Johns Hopkins University Press.

Martin, R. J., and Whitehouse, P. J. (1990). The clinical care of patients with dementia. In N. L. Mace, ed., *Dementia Care: Patient, Family, and Community,* pp. 22–31. Baltimore: Johns Hopkins University Press.

Maslow, K. (1994). Current knowledge about special care units: findings of a study by the U.S. Office of Technology Assessment. *Alzheimer Disease and Associated Disorders: An International Journal,* 8 (suppl. 1):S14-S40.

Masur, D. M., Sliwinski, M., Lipton, R. B., Blau, H. A., and Crystal, H. A. (1994). Neuropsychological prediction of dementia and the absence of dementia in healthy elderly person. *Neurology,* 44:1427–32.

Mayeux, R., Stern, Y., Ottman, R., et al. (1993). The apolipoprotein e4 allele in patients with Alzheimer's disease. *Annals of Neurology,* 34:752–54.

McGowin, D. F. (1993). *Living in the Labyrinth: A Personal Journey Through the Maze of Alzheimer's.* San Francisco: Elder Books.

McNeill, J. T. (1951). *A History of the Care of Souls.* New York: Harper & Brothers.

Meilaender, G. (1991). I want to burden my loved ones. *First Things,* 16 (October):12–16.

Meilaender, G. (1993). Terra es animata: on having a life. *Hastings Center Report,* 23(4):25–32.

Meleis, A. I., and Jonsen, A. R. (1983). Ethical crises and cultural differences. *Western Journal of Medicine,* 138:889-93.

Michelson, C., Mulvihill, M., Hsu, M., and Olson, E. (1991). Eliciting medical care preferences from nursing home residents. *Gerontologist,* 31:358–63.

Miles, S. (1991). Informed demand for "non-beneficial" medical treatment. *New England Journal of Medicine,* 325:26–28.

Miller, F. G., Quill, T. E., Brody, H., Fletcher, J. C., Gostin, L. O., and Meier, D. E. (1994). Regulating physician-assisted death. *New England Journal of Medicine,* 331:119–23.

Miller, R. J. (1992). Hospice care as an alternative to euthanasia. *Law, Medicine and Health Care,* 20:127–32.

Moody, H. R. (1992). *Ethics in an Aging Society.* Baltimore: Johns Hopkins University Press.

Morishita, L. (1990). Wandering behavior. In J. L. Cummings and B. L. Miller, eds., *Alzheimer's Disease: Treatment and Long-Term Management,* pp. 157–76. New York: Marcel Dekker.

Morris, J. C., ed. (1994). *Handbook of Dementing Illnesses.* New York: Marcel Dekker.

Mullan, M., Houldèn, H., Windelspecht, M., et al. (1992). A major locus for familial early onset Alzheimer's disease is on the long arm of chromosome 14, proximal to alpha-antichymotrypsin. *Nature Genetics,* 2:340–42.

Muller-Hill, B. (1988). *Murderous Science: Elimination by Scientific Selection of Jews, Gypsies, and Others, Germany 1933-1945.* G. R. Fraser, trans. New York: Oxford University Press.

Naruse, S., Igarashi, S., Kobayashi, T., et al. (1991). Mis-sense mutation Val-Ile in exon 17 of amyloid precursor protein gene in Japanese familial Alzheimer's disease. *Lancet,* 337:978–79.

Nietzsche, F. (1968). *Twilight of the Idols/The Anti-Christ.* R. J. Hollingdale, trans. New York: Penguin Books.

Nolan, K., and Swenson, S. (1988). New tools, new dilemmas: genetic frontiers. *Hastings Center Report,* 18(5):40–46.

Nygren, A. (1982). *Agape and Eros.* P. S. Watson, trans. Chicago: University of Chicago Press.

In re O'Connor, 72 N.Y.2d 517, 531 N.E.2d 607, 534 N.Y.S.2d 889 (1988).

Okin, S. M. (1989). *Justice, Gender, and the Family.* New York: Basic Books.

Palmer, R. E. (1969). *Hermeneutics.* Chicago: Northwestern University Press.

Patel, V., and Hope, T. (1993). Aggressive behavior in elderly people with dementia: a review. *International Journal of Geriatric Psychiatry,* 8:457–72.

Pearlman, R. A., and Uhlmann, R. F. (1988). Quality of life in chronic diseases perceptions of elderly patients. *Journal of Gerontology: Medical Sciences,* 43:25–30.

Pellegrino, E. D., and Thomasma, D. C. (1988). *For the Patient's Good: The Restoration of Beneficence in Health Care.* New York: Oxford University Press.

Percival, T. (1849). *Medical Ethics.* Oxford: John Henry Parker.

Pifer, A., and Bronte, L., ed. (1986). *Our Aging Society: Paradox and Promise.* New York: W. W. Norton.

Podolsky, D. (1992). New drugs for once unyielding diseases. *U.S. News & World Report;* 10 May, 67–68.

Porter, R. (1989). *A Social History of Madness: The World Through the Eyes of the Insane.* New York: E. P. Dutton.

Post, S. G. (1990a). Women and elderly parents: moral controversy in an aging society. *Hypatia: A Journal of Feminist Philosophy,* 5 (1):83–89.

Post, S. G. (1990b). Severely demented elderly people: a case against senicide. *Journal of the American Geriatrics Society,* 38:715–18.

Post, S. G. (1993a). *Inquiries in Bioethics.* Washington, D.C.: Georgetown University Press.

Post, S .G. (1993b). Tension between person and community. In R. A. Kane and A. L. Caplan, eds. *Ethical Conflicts in the Management of Home Care: The Case Manager's Dilemma,* pp. 101–8. New York: Springer Publishing.

Post, S. G. (1994). *Spheres of Love: Toward a New Ethics of the Family.* Dallas: Southern Methodist University Press.

Post, S. G., Botkin, J. R., and Whitehouse, P. J. (1992). Selective abortion for familial Alzheimer disease? *Obstetrics And Gynecology,* 79:794–98.

Post, S. G., and Leisey, R. G. (1995). Analogy, evaluation, and moral disagreement. *Journal of Value Inquiry,* 29:45–55.

Prado, C. G. (1990). *The Last Choice: Preemptive Suicide in Advanced Age.* New York: Greenwood Press.

Protzman, F. (1989). Killing of 49 elderly patients by nurse aids stuns Austria. *New York Times,* 18 April:1A.

Quill, T. E. (1993). *Death and Dignity: Making Choices and Taking Charge.* New York: W. W. Norton.

Quill, T. E., Cassel, C. K., and Meier, D. E. (1992). Care of the hopelessly ill: proposed clinical criteria for physician-assisted suicide. *New England Journal of Medicine,* 327:1380–84.

Ramsey, P. (1970). *The Patient as Person.* New Haven: Yale University Press.

Randall, J. H. (1926). *The Making of the Modern Mind: A Survey of the Intellectual Background of the Present Age.* Boston: Houghton Mifflin.

Rango, N. (1985). The nursing home resident with dementia: clinical care ethics, and policy considerations. *Annals of Internal Medicine,* 102:835–41.

Reifler, B. V., Henry, R. S., and Sherrill, K. A. (1992). A national demonstration program on dementia day care centers and respite services: an interim report. *Behavior, Health and Aging,* 2:199–206.

Reuben, D. B., Silliman, R. A., and Traines, M. (1988). The aging driver: medicine, policy and ethics. *Journal of The American Geriatrics Society,* 36:1135–42.

Rice, D. P., Fox, P. J., Max, W., et al. (1993). The economic burden of Alzheimer's disease care. *Health Affairs,* 12 (2):164–76.

Richman, J. (1992). A rational approach to rational suicide. In A. A. Leenaars, R. W. Maris, J. L. McIntosh, and J. Richman, eds., *Suicide and the Older Adult,* pp. 130–41. New York: Guilford Press.

Riley, K. P. (1989). Psychological interventions in Alzheimer's disease. In G. C. Gilmore, P. J. Whitehouse, and M. L. Wykle, eds., *Memory, Aging & Dementia,* pp. 199–211. New York: Springer Publishing

Ripich, D., and Wykle, M. (1990). Developing health care professionals' communication skills with Alzheimer's disease patients. Paper presented at the annual meeting of the American Society on Aging, San Francisco.

Roses, A., Pericak-Vance, M., Alberts, M., Saunders, A., Taylor, H., Gilbert, J., Schwartbach, C., Peacock, M., Fink, J., Bhasin, R., and Goldgaber, D. (1992). Locus heterogeneity of Alzheimer's disease. In F. Boller, F. Forette, Z. Khachaturian, M. Poncet, and Y. Christen, eds., *Heterogeneity of Alzheimer's Disease,* pp. 101–17. Berlin: Springer-Verlag.

Rothman, B. K. (1986). *The Tentative Pregnancy: Prenatal Diagnosis and the Future of Motherhood.* New York: Penguin Books.

Sabat, S. R., and Harre, R. (1992). The construction and deconstruction of self in Alzheimer's disease. *Ageing and Society,* 12:443–61.

Salzman, C. (1985). Clinical guideline for the use of antidepressant drugs in geriatric patients. *Clinical Psychiatry,* 46(10):38–43.

Satlin, A., Volicer, L., and Ross, V. (1992). Bright light treatment of behavioral and sleep disturbances in patients with Alzheimer's disease. *American Journal of Psychiatry,* 148:1028–32.

Saunders, A. M., Strittmatter, W. J., Schmechel, D., et al. (1993). Association of apolipoprotein E allele 4 with late-onset familial and sporadic Alzheimer's disease. *Neurology,* 43:1467–72.

Savishinsky, J. S. (1992). Intimacy, domesticity and pet therapy with the elderly: expectation and experience among nursing home volunteers. *Social Science and Medicine,* 34:1325–34.

Schellenberg, G. D., Bird, T. D., Wijsman, E. M., et al. (1992). Genetic linkage evidence for a familial Alzheimer's disease locus on chromosome 14. *Science,* 258:668–71.

Sehgal, A., Galbraith, A., Chesney, M., Schoenfeld, P., Charles, G., and Lo, B. (1992). How strictly do dialysis patients want their advance directives followed? *Journal of the American Medical Association,* 267:59–63.

Selkoe, D. J. (1992). Alzheimer's disease: new insights into an emerging epidemic. *Journal of Geriatric Psychiatry,* 25:211–27.

Shapiro, E., and Tate, R. B. (1985). Predictors of long-term care facility use among the elderly. *Canadian Journal of Aging,* 4:11–19.

Sidgwick, H. (1981 [original 1907]). *The Methods of Ethics.* Indianapolis: Hackett Publishing.

Simmel, G. (1950). *The Sociology of Georg Simmel.* K. H. Wolkff, ed. New York: Free Press.

Singer, P. (1993). *Practical Ethics.* New York: Cambridge University Press.

Skolnick, A., and Skolnick, J. H. (1980). *Family in Transition.* Boston: Little, Brown.

Slote, M. A. (1979). Obedience and illusions. In O. O'Neill and W. Ruddick, eds., *Having Children: Philosophical and Legal Reflections on Parenthood,* pp. 319–26. New York: Oxford University Press.

Smith, D. H. (1992). Seeing and knowing dementia. In R. H. Binstock, S. G. Post, and P. J. Whitehouse, eds., *Dementia and Aging: Ethics, Values, and Policy Choices,* pp. 44–54. Baltimore: Johns Hopkins University Press.

Soble, A. (1990). *The Structure of Love.* New Haven: Yale University Press.

Solomon, K., and Szwabo, P. (1992). Psychotherapy for patients with dementia. In J. E. Morley, R. M. Coe, R. Strong, and G. T. Grossberg, eds., *Memory Function and Aging-Related Disorders,* pp. 295–319. New York: Springer Publishing.

Sommers, C. H. (1986). Filial morality. *Journal of Philosophy,* 83 (8):439–56.

Spanjer, M. (1994). Mental suffering as justification for euthanasia in the Netherlands. *Lancet,* 343:1630.

Spar, J. E., and LaRue, A. (1990). *Geriatric Psychiatry.* Washington, D.C.: American Psychiatric Press.

St. George-Hyslop, P. H., Haines, J. L., Farrer, L. A., et al. (1990). Genetic linkage studies suggest that Alzheimer's disease is not a single homogeneous disorder. *Nature* 347:194–97.

St. George-Hyslop, P. H., Tanzi, R. E., Polinske, R. J., et al. (1987). The genetic defect causing familial Alzheimer's disease maps on chromosome 21. *Science* 235:885–890.

State of California, Title 17, California Code of Regulations, Section 2572, Chapter 321, Statutes of 1987, amending Section 410 of the Health and Safety Code.

Strittmatter, W. J., Saunders, A. M., Schmechel, D., Pericak-Vance, M., Enghild, J., Salvesen, G. S., and Roses, A. D. (1993). Apolipoprotein E: high-avidity binding to beta-amyloid and increased frequency of type 4 allele in late-onset familial Alzheimer disease. *Proceedings of the National Academy of Sciences,* 90:1977–81.

Sullivan, R. J. (1993). Accepting death without artificial nutrition or hydration. *Journal of General Internal Medicine,* 8:220–24.

Swift, J. (1945; 1727 original). *Gulliver's Travels.* Garden City, N. Y.: Doubleday.

Swift, J. (1993). *Selected Poems.* P. Rogers, ed. London: Penguin Books.

Tarnas, R. (1991). *The Passion of the Western Mind: Understanding the Ideas That Have Shaped Our World View.* New York: Ballantine Books.

Taylor, C. (1989). *The Sources of the Self: The Making of the Modern Identity.* Cambridge, Mass.: Harvard University Press.

Teichmann, J. (1985). The definition of person. *Philosophy,* 60(232):175–85.

Teri, L., Larson, E. B., and Reifler, B. V. (1988). Psychiatric phenomena in Alzheimer's disease. *Journal of the American Geriatrics Society,* 36:1–6.

Teri, L., and Logsdon, R. (1990). Assessment and management of behavioral disturbances in Alzheimer's disease. *Comprehensive Therapy,* 16(5):36–42.

Teri, L., Rabins, P., Whitehouse, P. J., Berg, L., Reisberg, B., Sunderland, T., Eichelman, B., and Phelps, C. (1992). Management of behavior disturbance in Alzheimer's disease: current knowledge and future directions. *Alzheimer Disease and Associated Disorders: An International Journal,* 6:77–88.

Thomasma, D. C. (1989). Moving the aged into the house of the dead: a critique of ageist social policy. *Journal of the American Geriatrics Society,* 37:169–72.

Thomasma, D.C. (1991). From ageism toward autonomy. In R. H. Binstock, S. G. Post, eds., *Too Old for Health Care? Controversies in Medicine, Law, Economics, and Ethics,* pp. 138–63. Baltimore: Johns Hopkins University Press.

Tillich, P. (1952). *The Courage to Be.* New Haven: Yale University Press.

Tomlinson, T., and Brody, H. (1990). Futility and the ethics of resuscitation. *Journal of the American Medical Association,* 264:1276–78.

Tooley, M. (1983). *Abortion and Infanticide.* Oxford: Clarendon Press.

Tribe, L. H. (1978). *American Constitutional Law.* Mineola, N. Y.: Foundation Press.

Truog, R. D., Berde, C. B., Mitchell, C., and Grier, H. E. (1992). Barbiturates in the care of the terminally ill. *New England Journal of Medicine,* 327:1678–82.

Truog, R. D., Brett, A. S., Frader, J. (1992). The problem with futility. *New England Journal of Medicine,* 326:1560–64.

Tucker, D. M., Watson, R. T., and Heilman, K. M. (1977). Affective discrimination and evocation in patients with right parietal disease. *Neurology*, 17:947–50.

U.S. Congress Office of Technology Assessment (1987). *Losing a Million Minds: Confronting the Tragedy of Alzheimer's Disease and Other Dementias* (OTA-BA-323). Washington, D.C.: Office of Technology Assessment.

U.S. Congress Office of Technology Assessment (1992). *Special Care Units for People with Alzheimer's and Other Dementias*. Washington, D.C.: U.S. Government Printing Office.

Volicer, L. (1986). Need for hospice approach to treatment of patients with advanced progressive dementia. *Journal of the American Geriatrics Association*, 34: 655–58.

Walter, J. J., and Shannon, T. A., eds. (1990). *Quality of Life: The New Medical Dilemma*. New York: Paulist Press.

Weaver, G. D. (1986). Senile dementia and resurrection theology. *Theology Today*, 42(4):444–56.

Wechsler, J. J. (1993). The view of rabbinic literature. In L. M. Cohen, ed. *Justice Across Generations: What Does It Mean?*, pp. 19–34. Washington, D. C.: American Association of Retired Persons.

Wertz, D. C., and Fletcher, J. C. (1989). Fatal knowledge? prenatal diagnosis and sex selection. *Hastings Center Report*, 19(3):21–27.

Whitehouse, P. J., ed. (1993). *Dementia*. Philadelphia: F. A. Davis.

Wildes, K. W., ed. (1994). *Journal of Medicine and Philosophy*, 19(2).

Williams, S. (1993). Revolutionizing the genetics of Alzheimer's disease. *Research and Practice* (published by the national Alzheimer's Association), 2(2):1–2.

World Federation of Neurology: Research Committee Research Group on Huntington's Chorea. (1989). Ethical issues policy statement on Huntington's disease molecular genetics predictive test. *Journal of Neurological Sciences*, 94:327–32.

Wright, L. K. (1993). *Alzheimer's Disease and Marriage: An Intimate Account*. Newbury Park, Calif.: SAGE Publications.

Wyschogrod, E. (1990). *Saints and Postmodernism: Revisioning Moral Philosophy*. Chicago: University of Chicago Press.

Zgola, J. M. (1987). *Doing Things: A Guide to Programming Activities for Persons with Alzheimer's Disease and Related Disorders*. Baltimore: Johns Hopkins University Press.

Zweibel, N. R., and Cassel, C. K. (1989). Treatment choices at the end of life: a comparison of decisions by older patients and their physician-selected proxies. *Gerontologist*, 29:615–21.

❧ Index

About the Author

STEPHEN G. POST received a Ph.D. degree in ethics from the University of Chicago Divinity School. He is currently associate professor in the Center for Biomedical Ethics of the School of Medicine, Case Western Reserve University, where he also holds appointments in the Departments of Philosophy and Religion. Post is an elected Fellow of the Hastings Center and a senior Research Fellow of the Kennedy Institute of Ethics at Georgetown University.

Post served as associate editor for the second edition of the *Encyclopedia of Bioethics* (five volumes, 1995). His most recent books include *Inquiries in Bioethics* (1993) and *Spheres of Love: Toward a New Ethics of the Family* (1994). He coedited *Dementia and Aging: Ethics, Values, and Policy Choices* (Johns Hopkins University Press, 1992).

Library of Congress Cataloging-in-Publication Data

Post, Stephen Garrard, 1951–
    The moral challenge of Alzheimer disease / Stephen G. Post.
        p.   cm.
    Includes bibliographical references and index.
    ISBN 0-8018-5174-2 (hc : alk. paper)
        1. Alzheimer's disease—Moral and ethical aspects.   I. Title.
RC523.P67   1996
362.1'96831—dc20   95-13505